AQUA TONE

AQUATIC STRENGTH TRAINING

**Stronger Muscles
Less Stress
In the Water**

**BY
PATTY BOWMAN**

Outskirts Press, Inc.
Denver, Colorado

The opinions expressed in this manuscript are solely the opinions of the author and do not represent the opinions or thoughts of the publisher. The author has represented and warranted full ownership and/or legal right to publish all the materials in this book.

Aqua Tone
Aquatic Strength Training
All Rights Reserved.
Copyright © 2008 Patty Bowman
V3.0

This book may not be reproduced, transmitted, or stored in whole or in part by any means, including graphic, electronic, or mechanical without the express written consent of the publisher except in the case of brief quotations embodied in critical articles and reviews.

Outskirts Press, Inc.
http://www.outskirtspress.com

ISBN: 978-1-4327-1090-3

Outskirts Press and the "OP" logo are trademarks belonging to Outskirts Press, Inc.

PRINTED IN THE UNITED STATES OF AMERICA

INTRODUCTION

At some point while I was teaching Aqua Aerobics, I decided that I would enjoy working with people on a smaller scale based on their goals and progress. This was my first step into the world of Personal Training. I discovered that the Aquatic Exercise Association (AEA) offered an Aquatic Personal Training certification. I knew that I would have to fly out of Alaska to get this certification so I felt I should talk to our Fitness Manager, Donna Fisher, first and see if she saw a place for this in our health club. Her response was positive, but she would require that I complete a land personal training program first. As a result I became certified through the Aerobics and Fitness Association of America (AFAA) as a Personal Trainer. In the fall of 2003, I flew to Omaha, Nebraska to participate in the AEA Aquatic Personal Training Certification course and received the prize for traveling the farthest distance for the class.

After returning, I began to work and learn with Donna about weight training on land. I also started experimenting with resistance equipment in the water. I used already tried and true exercises and equipment, but also began to experiment with coated free weights, rubber tubing and ankle weights. I was becoming intrigued with the many ways we might find to create strength training in the water. It was fun to apply land principles to the water and discover the ways these principles are similar and different with regards to the type of equipment and movement in these two environments.

At this time, one of our other Personal Trainers, Patricia Davis, approached me about the need for a water class for resistance training. She was the catalyst for taking it to the next step. This is how Aqua Tone started. It took us a year to put our program together. We had to find times to meet (busy schedules on both our parts), perform the exercises, experiment with differing types of equipment, and utilize the space, depth and anchor points available in our pool. It took us another year of promoting and fine tuning our program to fit the needs of our health club and satisfy the expectations of our managers. However, it finally became a reality and I believe a successful addition to our club and members.

Teaching the class has and will continue to teach me. By this I mean that I am learning from watching and listening to the participants. What works for one may not work for another. Knowing this I revise or adapt if necessary. However, the fundamentals stay the same. Proper form and body mechanics are essential. Creatively trying new ideas that are safe and effective continues to be fun and exciting.

"Do not follow where the path may lead
Go instead where there is no path
And leave a trail."

Ralph Waldo Emerson
1803-1882
American Poet

ACKNOWLEDGMENTS

I extend my MANY thanks to:

- **Patricia Davis for the vision she had for the program and dedication to co-creating it with me.**
- **Donna Fisher who has been my teacher and mentor.**
- **Janet Cenker and Mary Bunten, my aqua friends and co-teachers, who have been so supportive of this program.**
- **Loyola McManus for a genuine willingness to share her time and professional expertise.**
- **Sheila Bratten for her beauty and poise for the pictures in this book**
- **Martha Markey for giving me inspiration and direction in writing and publishing**
- **My family, Keith, Will and Melissa for their technological support in creating this book.**
- **The Aqua Tone participants who continue to teach me through their attendance and feedback.**
- **AEA and AFAA for their professional education and certifications**
- **The Alaska Club/Fairbanks for giving me the opportunity and facilities to create this program.**
- **Finally, <u>but most important</u>, to God for creating the waters!**

"If I'd known I was gonna live this long
I'd have taken better care of myself."

Eubie Blake (at age 100)
1883-1983
American Songwriter/Composer

PREFACE

My goals for this book were to:

- Increase the awareness of possibilities of resistance training in the water both for aqua teachers, personal trainers and individuals.

- Provide knowledge about proper body form, exercise technique and general resistance training principles to facilitate the design of a safe and effective program.

- Keep the format simple

The information in this book is, of course, not all inclusive. There may be variations that a knowledgeable person can apply or there may be adaptations needed based on physical differences or needs.

It is important to note that each exercise should be considered with regard to its safety for individual concerns and health status. Participants should consult a Physician when beginning any exercise program if there are health conditions or risks. The water can sometimes be the best place to start for those who have injuries, chronic pain, health conditions or are just starting an exercise program.

IT IS A PROVEN FACT THAT RESISTANCE TRAINING BUILDS STRONGER MUSCLES AND BONES. I dedicate this book to those of you, like myself, who love and believe in the conditioning, training and therapeutic effects of the water AND LOVE TO BE IN IT! WHY NOT TRY IT?

"If you don't do what's best for your body
You're the one who comes up on the short end."

Julius Erving (Dr. J)
American Basketball Player

TABLE OF CONTENTS

Terms to Know	**11-12**
Aquatone Defined	**15**
Aquatone Program	**19-23**
Aquatone Equipment	**27-34**
Aquatone Exercises	**37-71**
Aquatone Stretching	**74-75**
References	**77-78**
Author Information	**79**

"The only way to keep your health
Is to eat what you don't want
Drink what you don't like
And do what you'd druther not."

Mark Twain
1835-1910
American Writer/Humorist

Terms to know

Anterior – The front of the body or body part

Posterior – The back of the body or body part

Medial – Toward the midline of the left and right sides

Lateral – To the side, away from the midline

Hyperextend – To extend the joint of a body part beyond the normal range of motion.

Abduction – Movement of a limb away from the middle of the body

Adduction – Movement of a limb toward the middle of the body

Concentric – The hard part of an isotonic resistance movement in which the muscle shortens.

Eccentric – The easy part of an isotonic resistance movement in which the muscle lengthens while maintaining tension.

Isotonic Muscle Contraction – A movement in which the body part is moving against resistance and the muscle shortens as it contracts.

Warm Up - A 5-10 minute period of light exercise in which the muscles are warmed up in preparation for more vigorous exercise.

Cool Down – The final part of an exercise routine which gradually reduces the heart rate.

Neutral Wrist – The position of the wrist in which it makes a straight line between the elbow and the hand. It is neither flexed or hyperextended.

Neutral Shoulder - The natural position of the shoulder when standing with arms at side, palms facing body. The shoulder is not rotated in any manner.

Muscle Overload – In order to improve in muscular strength and endurance a person must work the muscle beyond its normal capacity to the point of fatigue or failure.

Progressive Overload - As the body adapts to a load it must be progressively challenged to see any further gains.

Training to failure – Continuing resistance until it is difficult or impossible to complete more repetitions.

Opposing muscle groups – Each muscle has an opposing muscle that performs the opposite movement. The major opposing muscle groups include the biceps/triceps, chest/back, abdominals/lower back, quadriceps/hamstrings.

Core muscles – These are the abdominal and back muscles that support the body. They include the Transverse Abdominus, External and Internal Obliques, Rectus Abdominus and Erector Spinae.

Target Muscle – This is the prime mover or primary muscle that is contracting during a resistance movement.

Assisting Muscle – These are muscles that assist the prime mover in a resistance movement. They are also called synergists.

Super Sets – An advanced programming technique in which two types of exercises are performed without rest in between.

Pyramiding/Triangles – An advanced programming technique in which the weight is increased or decreased with each set (Heavy to light or light to heavy).

Two-Hour Pain Rule –This is an arthritis term. The Arthritis Foundation states "If you have more arthritis pain two hours after exercising than you did before, you've probably done too much and should cut back a little."

THESE TERMS ARE UNDERLINED WITH AN ASTERISK IN THE TEXT SO THAT THE READER WILL KNOW TO REFER BACK FOR UNDERSTANDING THESE CONCEPTS.

AQUA TONE

DEFINED

"Health is worth more than learning."

Thomas Jefferson
1743-1826
3rd President of the United States

WHAT IS AQUA TONE?

Aqua Tone is aquatic resistance training using a variety of equipment to produce muscle overload* in major muscle groups and promote strength. Although there is an initial warm up with movement, exercises are mostly stationary and focused on resistance training rather than cardiovascular training. .

HOW IS MUSCLE OVERLOAD ACHIEVED IN THE WATER?

Muscle overload* can be achieved through increase in time, repetitions, force and speed or in the level of resistance, weight or drag.

WHY USE THE WATER?

The water provides natural resistance for strength training. With the addition of equipment, progressive muscular strength and endurance can be accomplished. However, the buoyancy of the water supports the muscles and joints, thus decreasing the chances of injury and strain. Since the forces of the water are pushing in all directions, a person has to work to stabilize the body thus engaging and strengthening core muscles.*

WHO MIGHT USE THIS PROGRAM?

Although this program is for anyone there are certain groups of individuals that this program may appeal to:

1. Average active person interested in changing up their work-out routine
2. De-conditioned individuals beginning a work-out program
3. Senior citizens
4. Individuals that either can't or won't use a regular weight room.
5. Those who love to work out in the water
6. Individuals with certain health risks or conditions. (With Doctor permission)
7. Post surgery/rehabilitation individuals (this should be done in cooperation with a doctor or a physical therapist)

"My goal has always been to help people help themselves.
Your body is your most priceless possession
You've got to take care of it."

Jack Lalanne
American Fitness/Exercise Expert

AQUA TONE

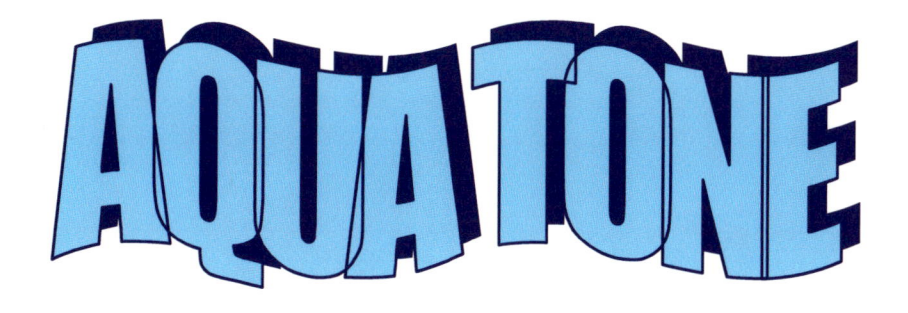

PROGRAM

"A man too busy to take care of his health
Is like a mechanic too busy to take care of his tools"

Spanish Proverb

PROGRAM GUIDELINES

Initially the participant should use light weight and learn and practice proper form and body mechanics for each exercise. If the individual is de-conditioned or recovering from injury it might be best to first use only the resistance of the water without equipment to perform the exercise. Increasing the level of resistance should be made as the participant feels that the target muscle* is unchallenged at the present level. Progression should be made using the methods mentioned earlier through increase in time, repetitions, force and speed or level of resistance, weight or drag.

After 6-8 weeks the participant can and should employ different programming techniques in order to stay challenged and to keep it interesting. This could be done through performing the exercises in a different order, adding new exercises or changing exercises for each muscle group. Other training methods such as supersets and pyramids* can be introduced and utilized by advanced participants.

When setting up a program follow these **American College of Sports Medicine (ACSM) recommendations** for resistance training:
1. Perform a minimum of 8-10 exercises that target and condition the major muscle groups (arms, shoulders, chest, abdomen, back, hips and legs)
2. Perform a minimum of 1 set of 8-12 repetitions OR to near failure.*
3. Perform resistance exercises 2-3 days per week. (not on consecutive days)

It is also important to create a program that targets opposing muscle groups* which trains them equally for muscle balance.

"Resistance training for the average participant should be rhythmical, performed at moderate to slow controlled speed, through a full range of motion and with a normal breathing pattern during the lifting movements."*

(* Quoted from The Recommended Quantity and Quality of Exercise for Developing and Maintaining Cardiorespiratory and Muscular Fitness and Flexibility in Healthy Adults, ACSM, Medicine and Science in Sports and Exercise, 1998)

PROGRAM FORMAT

There are many ways in which this program can be used and set up. It can be:

INDIVIDUAL PROGRAM
1. Choose exercises that are appropriate for skill and physical level
2. Consult ACSM guidelines
3. Consult Doctor if health conditions exist or arise

PERSONAL TRAINING PROGRAM
1. Choose exercises to meet individuals skill level and personal goals
2. Obtain medical clearance if health risks or conditions exist

CIRCUIT
1. Can be individual or group
2. Location of exercises depend on size, depth of pool, anchor points and available equipment
3. Allows individual instruction
4. Know limits and or restrictions for individuals

GROUP EXERCISE PROGRAM
1. Important to observe and correct improper body mechanics
2. Requires enough equipment so that all participants can experience progress and challenge.
3. Know limits and or restrictions for individuals in the group

Some sample exercise routines are given for individual and group programs on pages 70 and 71.

Our program is set up as a circuit. We do not have enough equipment for a group class and we also want to work with individuals more closely. The design and placement of our exercises are based on depth, anchor points and available space. There are 14 stations running for 3 minutes each. A picture of the exercise is placed at each station. We begin with a warm up time and end with a cool down and stretching. The class is set to music. The instructor is able to work with the group as well as each individual, teaching and correcting form if necessary.

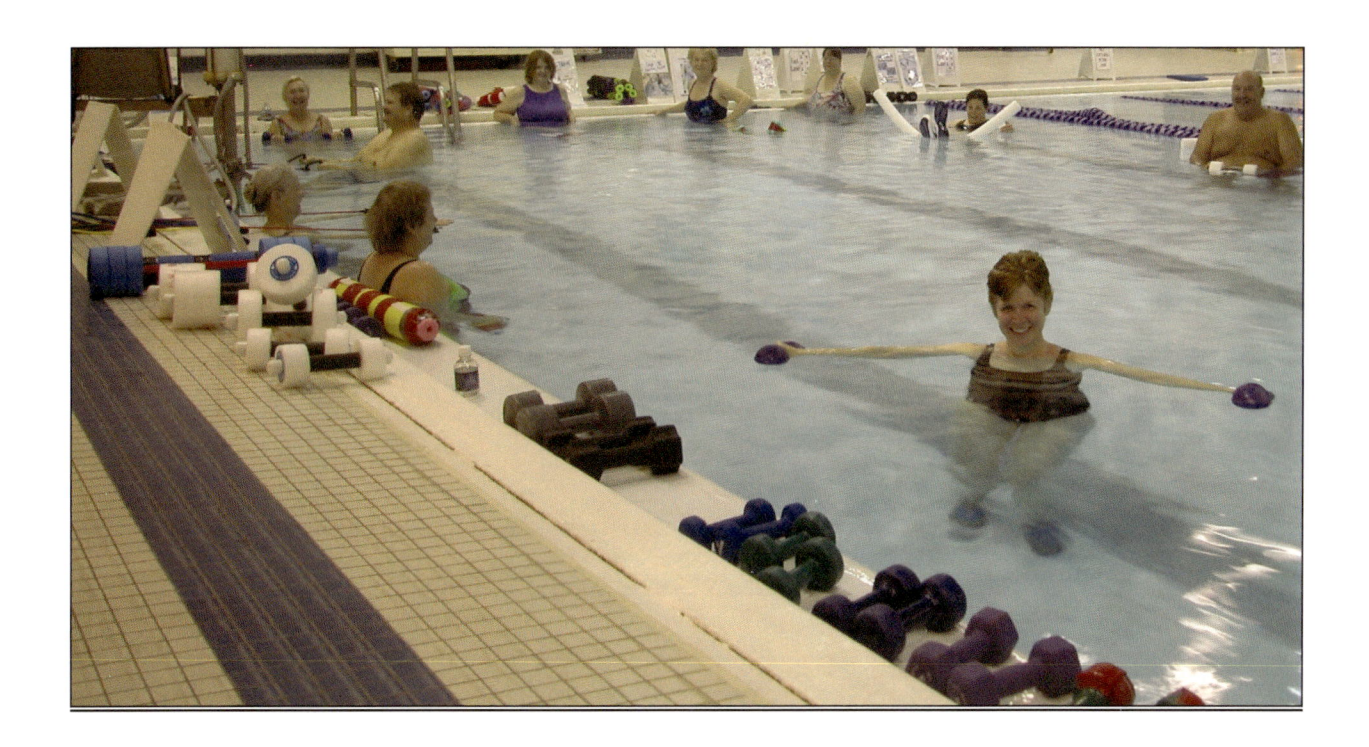

PROPER BODY FORM

Perform resistance exercises in neutral body position:

1. Shoulder blades are back and slightly down
2. Chest is slightly up and out
3. Chin is pulled slightly back and down
4. The natural arch in the lumbar and cervical regions of the spine is maintained.
5. Ears, shoulders, hips, knees and ankles are aligned.

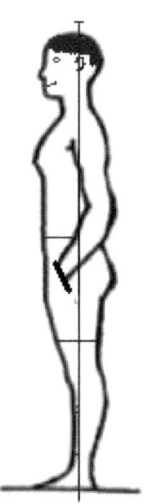

Maintaining this position reduces the risk of injury and increases the effectiveness of the movement or exercise for the target muscles.* Stabilization of the spine in this position also helps to strengthen the core muscles.* Certain abdominal exercises are the exception because the spine flexes to perform the exercise. Proper body form must be maintained at all times and not sacrificed for progress.

In the water:
1. The muscle that is being targeted should remain under the water while performing the movement
2. Water depth should allow for full range of motion under water surface

IMPORTANT PROGRAM CONSIDERATIONS

1. Always begin with a 5-10 minute warm-up* and end with a cool down.*
2. Stretch muscles after each exercise or at the end of the workout.
3. Keep muscles warm by jogging between sets.
4. Temperature of the water should be between 84-86 degrees   86 = 30°F
5. Keep in mind individual levels of ability and goals   83 =
6. Awareness of health or physical restrictions is imperative
7. Remember to breath during exercises (don't hold breath)
8. Charting progress is helpful and beneficial
9. Muscle soreness for a fatigued muscle is normal. **PAIN IN MUSCLES AND JOINTS IS NOT NORMAL.** Discontinue or decrease level of exercise for that muscle. Follow the Two-Hour Pain Rule* and seek medical advice if pain continues.
10. During the performance of each exercise, focus on the target muscle* and minimize body movement with the exception of the assisting muscles.*

---

*When the performance of an exercise becomes difficult and the muscles are becoming fatigued, there is a tendency to use other muscles to assist the effort. Pay attention to this and correct body form. If this is impossible, muscle failure has been achieved and the participant should stop performing the exercise for the current exercise session.

"He who enjoys good health is rich
Though he knows it not."

Italian Proverb

AQUA TONE

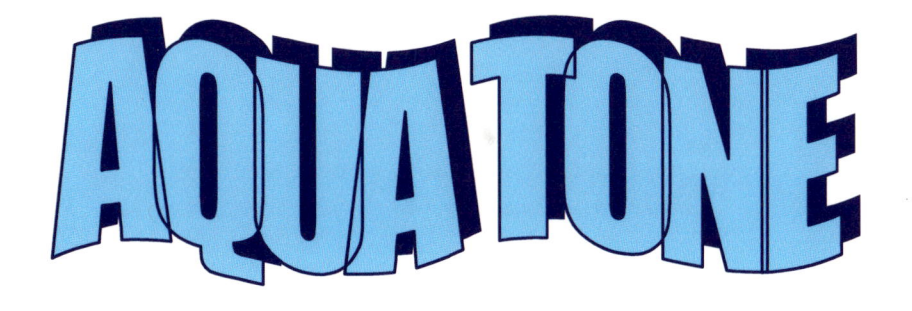

EQUIPMENT

"He who has health has hope
And he who has hope has everything."

Arabian Proverb

EQUIPMENT

Any equipment that is made of water compatible materials and has the capacity to be increased by weight, level of resistance or surface area can be used. However, an important concept to understand is that buoyancy affects muscle performance in a different way than land. Without equipment, all muscle actions in the water are concentric*. In the water the body is basically a piece of drag equipment. With the addition of equipment, concentric* and eccentric* muscle actions are dependent of the type of equipment. Following are some recommended types of equipment and the way muscle action is produced as a result of its type.

RUBBER TUBING

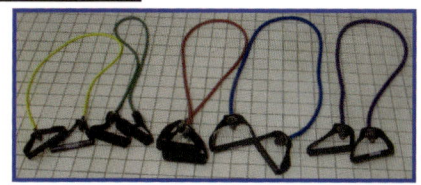

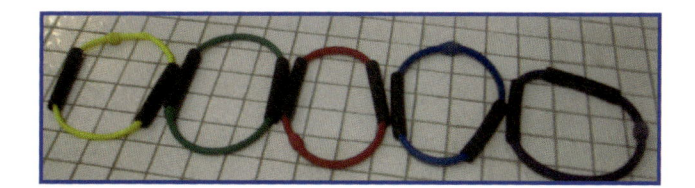

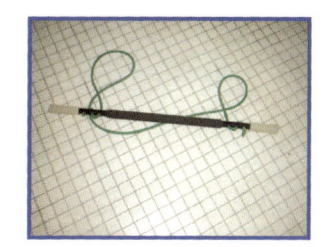

1. Resistance (concentric phase) is in the direction of the pull
2. Maintain control during eccentric phase
3. Check for cracks and wear. Replace for safety
4. Available in colors of progressive level of resistance

LATEX BANDS (CAN FIND NON-LATEX TYPES)

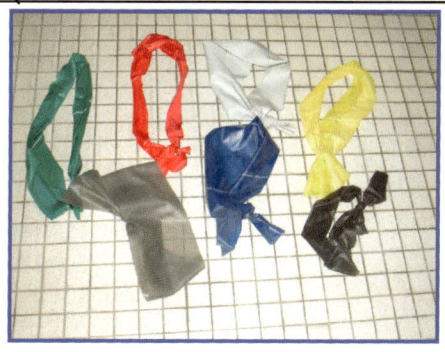

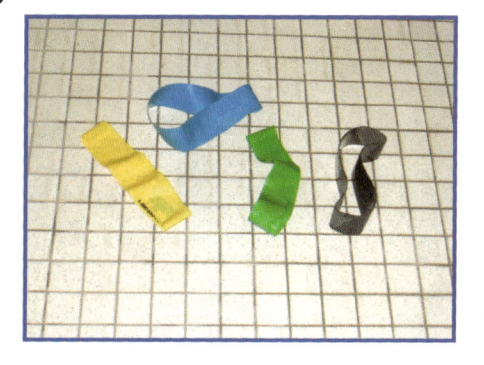

1. Resistance (concentric phase) is in the direction of the pull
2. Available in lengths that can be tied to create bands or purchased as bands
3. Available in colors of progressive level of resistance

FREE WEIGHTS

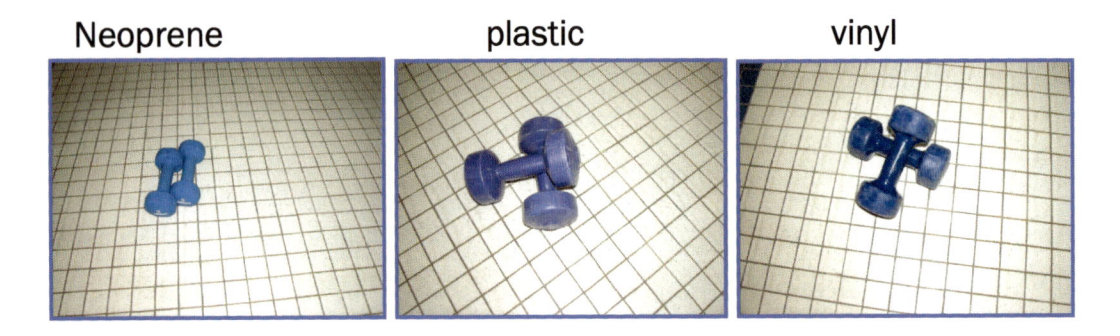

Neoprene · plastic · vinyl

1. Resistance (concentric phase) is upward
2. Maintain control during downward (eccentric) phase
3. Can be held and used to add body weight for certain exercises (i.e. for squats)
4. Available in progressive weights

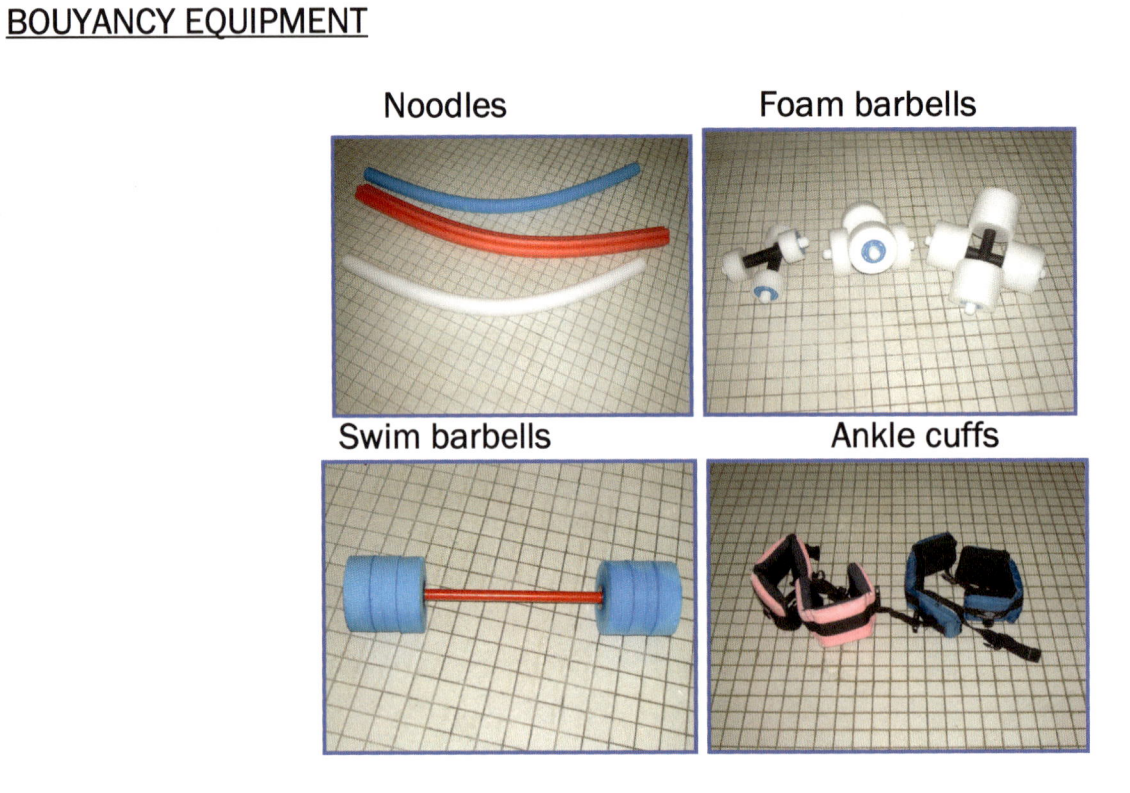

BOUYANCY EQUIPMENT

Noodles · Foam barbells

Swim barbells · Ankle cuffs

1. Resistance (concentric phase) is downward
2. Maintain control during upward (eccentric phase)
3. Adaptation needed for noodles to be progressive *

*SEE ADAPTED NOODLES

WEIGHTED ACCESSORIES

Weight vest

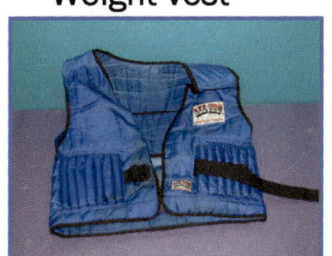

Ankle weights

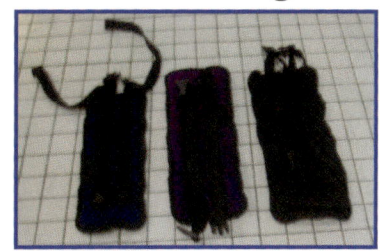

Diving Belt

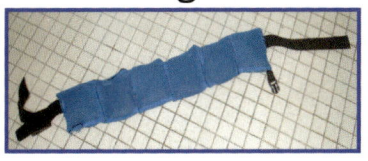

1. Resistance (concentric phase) is upward
2. Can add weight to pockets on most styles

DRAG EQUIPMENT

Gloves

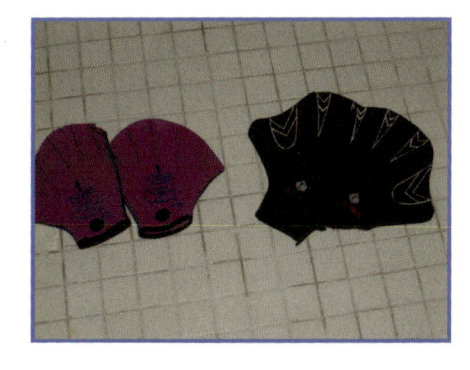

Fins

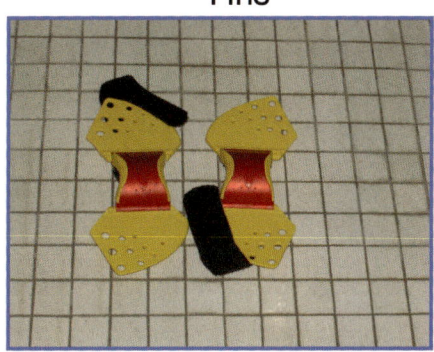

1. Resistance (concentric phase) is in both directions of movement
2. Good for beginning or therapy participants

OTHER

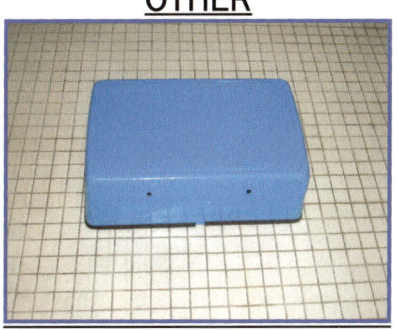

Aqua Step can be used for calf raises or interval step-ups.

CARE OF THE EQUIPMENT

The chlorine environment is very harsh on equipment especially those made out of latex and rubber. Here are some ideas to preserve your equipment.

1. After each use rinse/soak with cold water for a short time.
2. Dry it out (preferably away from the pool area).
3. Place rubber tubing in large plastic storage bags with zip lock closures after they are dry.
4. Heavy items such as weights can be stored in a closed container.
5. If metal weights are used to add weight to vests, belts, or ankle weights, be sure to dry the weights with a towel after use or wrap with a water proof covering to protect from rusting.

FINDING EQUIPMENT

First, check local stores such as sporting goods. Equipment can also be ordered from the following companies:

Aqua Fins
1 800 861-3211
AllegroMedical.com

Hydro-Fit
1 800 346-7295
hydrofit.com

Kiefer
1 800 323-4071
kiefer.com

Power Systems
1 800 321-6975
power-systems.com

Spri
1 800 222-7774
spriproducts.com

Thera-Band
1 800 321-2135
thera-band.com

Watergear
1 800 794-6432
watergear.com

ADAPTED NOODLES

The concept of progressive overload dictates that each exercise must have a method to continually increase the level of resistance. When setting up a resistance program for the water, equipment must be chosen for its ability to achieve this goal. Noodles are not progressive by nature and so following are some methods that we created in order to use them in the Aqua Tone program.

Materials that are needed might be varying sizes of noodles, straps, duct tape, scissors, sewing elastic, and a knife.

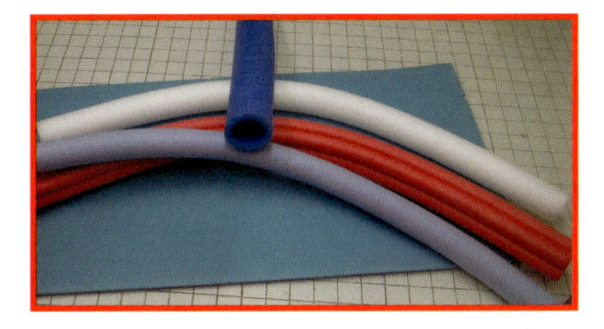

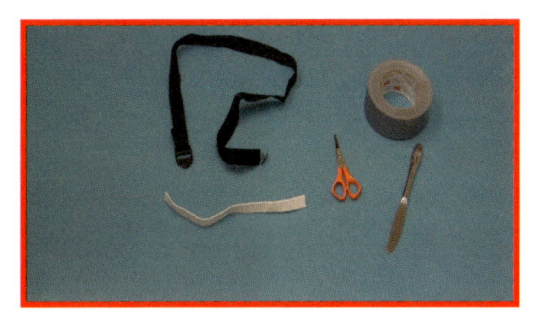

DUCT TAPE you say! How unprofessional you might be saying! Well, believe me it works very well. Some of our noodles have been used for more than a year in the water without being replaced. It is a marvel of modern technology.

FOR LEG NOODLES (Adduction, Hamstring curls, Quad pushdowns etc)

1. Cut a regular size noodle in half. Use a good solid noodle as this will be the base

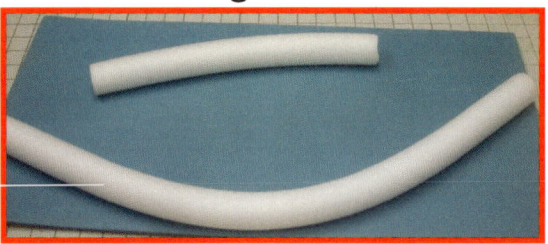

2. Cut smaller pieces from another noodle. These should be cut so that when placed on the ends of the longer noodle, there is a space in the middle for placing the foot.

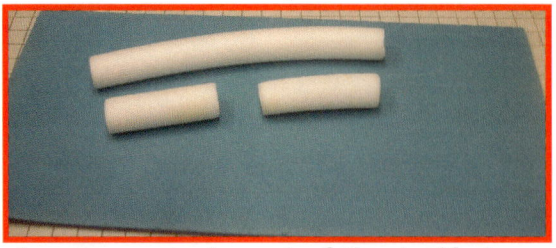

3. Strap or duct tape two pieces on each end of the half size noodle.

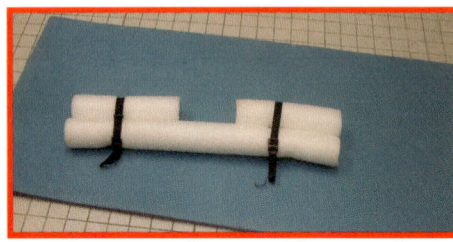

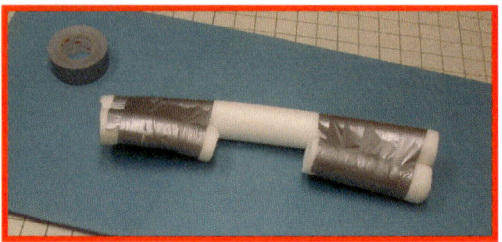

4. For progression, each noodle can have an added amount of pieces strapped or duct taped.

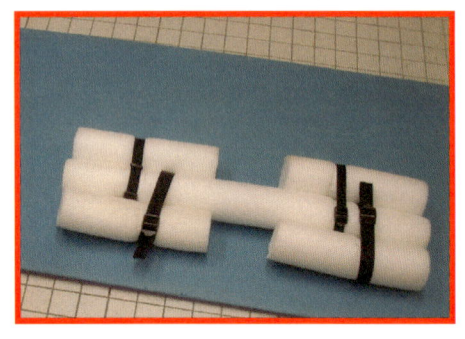

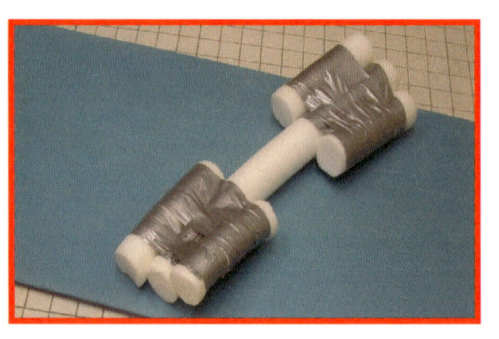

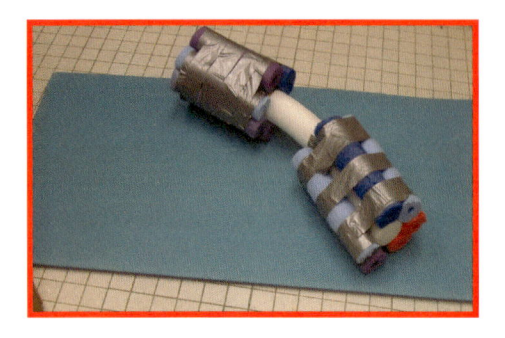

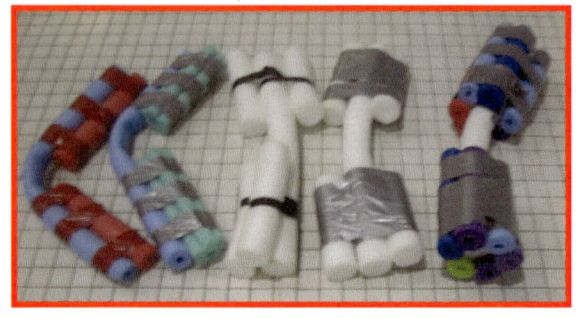

FOR ARMS (Triceps etc)

Method #1

1. Cut a noodle in half. Cut noodle with hole about four inches longer.

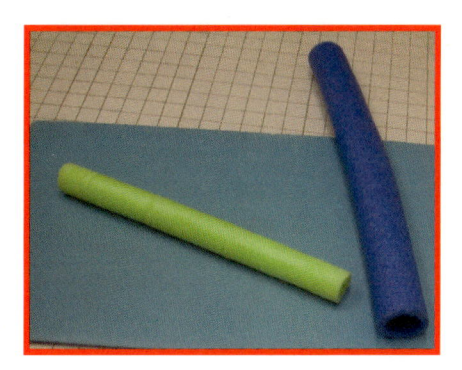

2. Place smaller noodle through hole. To get it all the way through use a twisting motion.

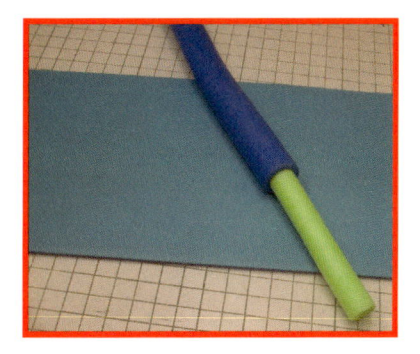

3. Duct tape 2 pieces of elastic on each side so that hands can slip into handles. Make sure that the handles are placed so that when the hands are slipped through they are lined up with the shoulders.

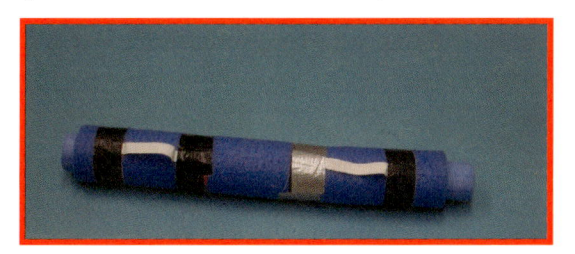

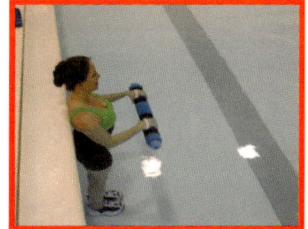

Method #2

1. Cut noodle in half. Use Styrofoam connectors.

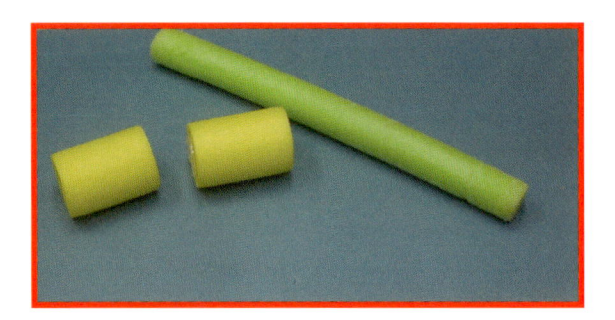

2. Add a connector to each end of the noodle. Duct tape on both sides to hold connectors in place. Otherwise connectors will pop off.

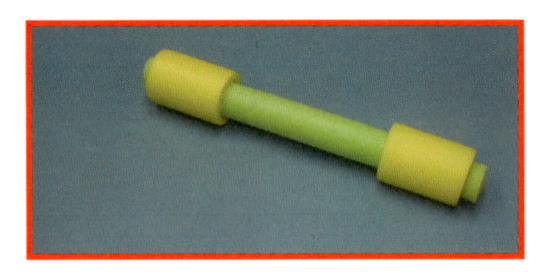

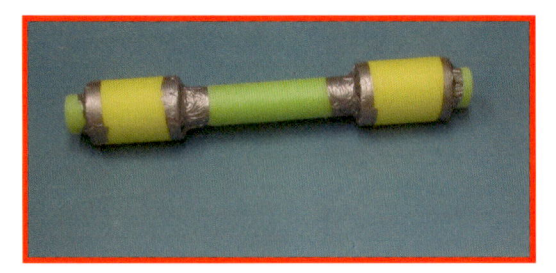

3. Duct tape elastic on both sides for handles.

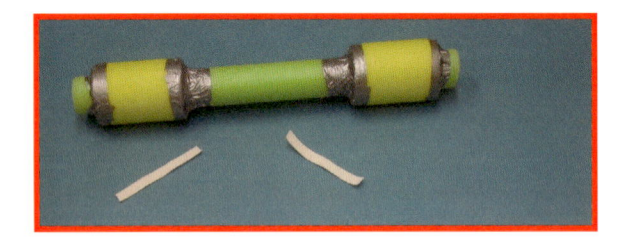

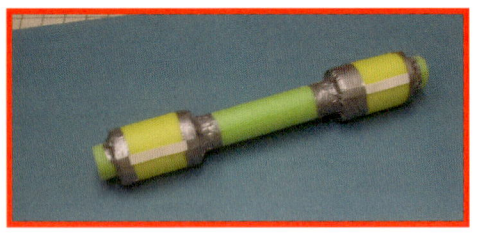

4. On a half noodle, four connectors can be used for increasing the resistance properties.

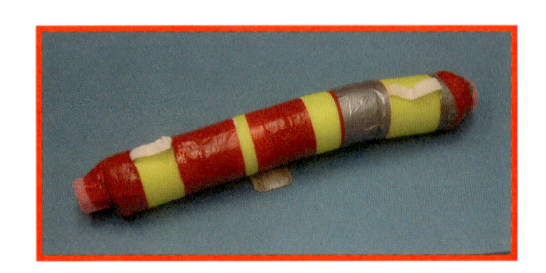

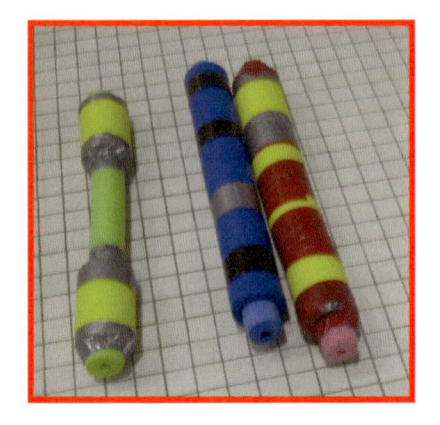

AQUA TONE

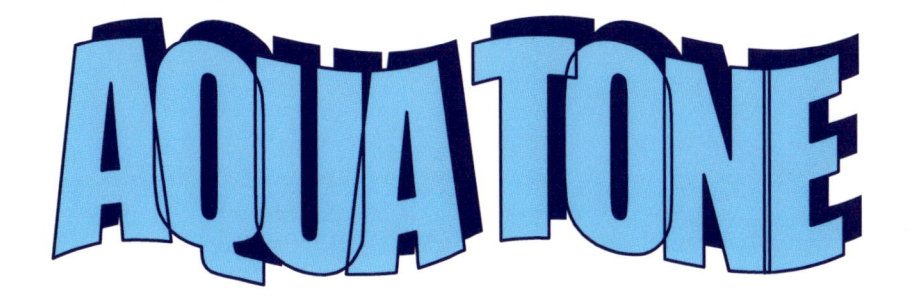

EXERCISES

"Physical fitness is not only one of the most important
Keys to a healthy body, it is the basis of
Dynamic and creative intellectual activity."

John F. Kennedy
1917-1963
35th President of the United States

Major Muscle Groups of the Human Body For Aqua Tone

(LifeART and Mediclip image copyright (2008) Wolters Kluwer Health, Inc. – Lippincott Williams & Wilkins. All Rights reserved.)

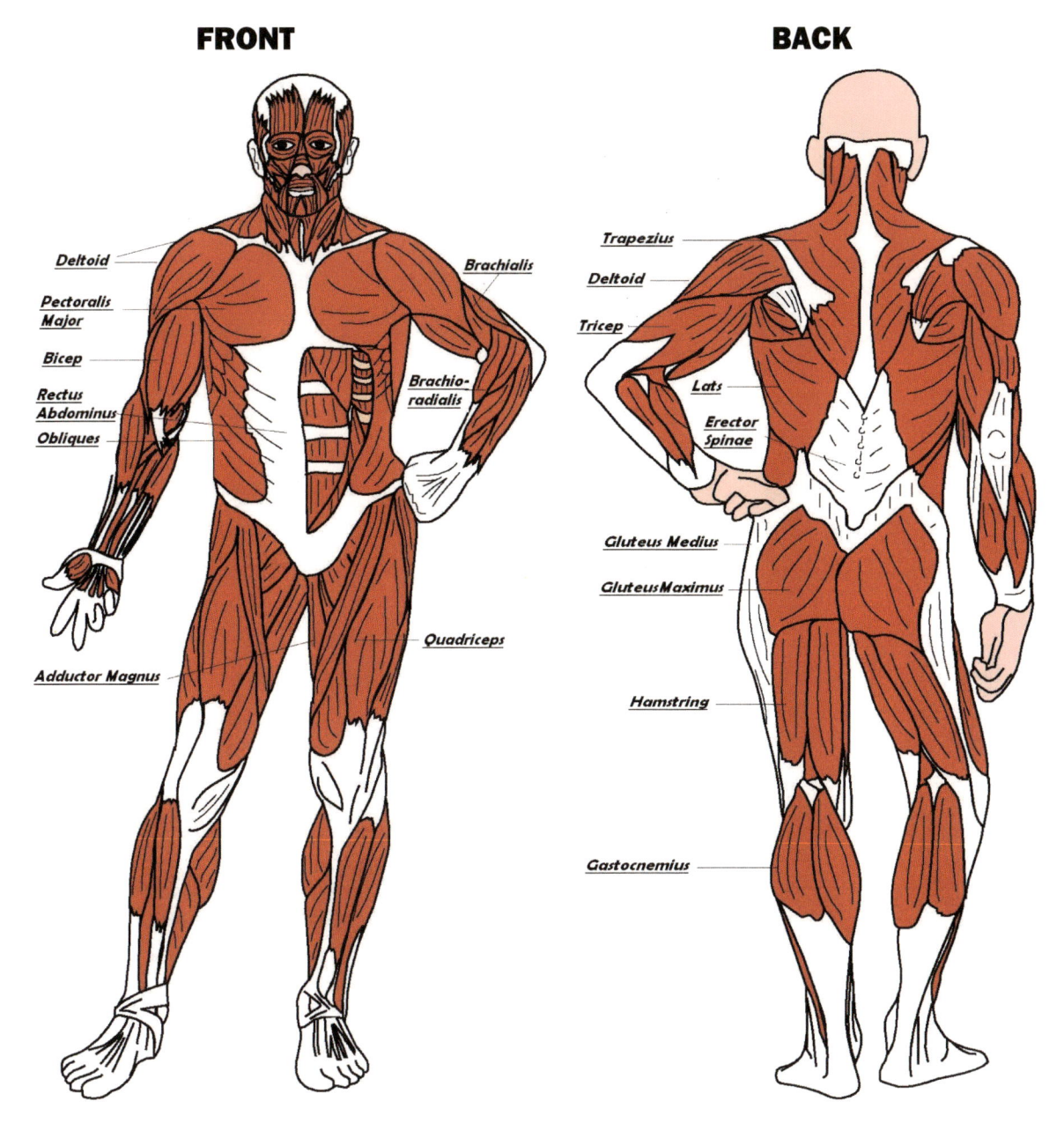

FRONT   **BACK**

Front labels: Deltoid, Pectoralis Major, Bicep, Rectus Abdominus, Obliques, Adductor Magnus, Brachialis, Brachioradialis, Quadriceps

Back labels: Trapezius, Deltoid, Tricep, Lats, Erector Spinae, Gluteus Medius, Gluteus Maximus, Hamstring, Gastocnemius

Deltoid = shoulder (anterior/medial)
Pectoralis Major = chest
Biceps = upper arm (front)
Brachialis = upper arm (side)
Brachioradialis = upper forearm
Rectus Abdominus = front length of torso
Obliques = both sides of torso
Adductor Magnus = inner thigh
Quadriceps = upper leg (front)

Deltoid = shoulder (posterior)
Trapezius = upper back
Tricep = upper arm (back)
Latissimus Dorsi = middle back
Erector Spinae = lower back
Gluteus Medius = hip
Gluteus Maximus = buttocks
Hamstrings = upper leg (back)
Gastrocnemius = calves

PERFORMING AND CHOOSING THE FOLLOWING EXERCISES

For each exercise the first picture and column give directions for the starting position. The second picture and column describe the way the exercise should be performed. Always return to the start position <u>completely</u> before progressing to the next repetition. It is important to read and perform these carefully for the exercise to be safe and effective. General reminders are in red. Cautions are in red but also capitalized to stress their importance.

Only the focus <u>target muscles</u>* are named. However, during the execution of an exercise <u>assisting muscles</u>* are at work. For example, the target muscles for the compound row are the latissimus dorsi and the posterior deltoids. The biceps would also be involved in the pulling motion so there may be some soreness or feelings of work and overall improvement for these muscles as well.

REMEMBER:

1. Choose the exercises and equipment that are appropriate for skill level (beginner to advanced) and health status. These levels are outlined on page 70. Consult a Physician if necessary.
2. Identify any physical restrictions and or problem areas (shoulders, neck, back, hips, knees etc). Choose exercises accordingly and follow any special guidelines or cautions.
3. Follow PROGRAM GUIDELINES in program chapter:

    - ✓ Start light and learn the proper form and technique for each exercise
    - ✓ Progress according to present conditioning level, physical restrictions and or health status
    - ✓ Change it up every 6-8 weeks
    - ✓ Follow ACSM guidelines for creating your routine

AQUA TONE

LATERAL RAISES / PULL DOWNS Target Muscles: Medial Deltoids
Latissimus Dorsi

HANDS

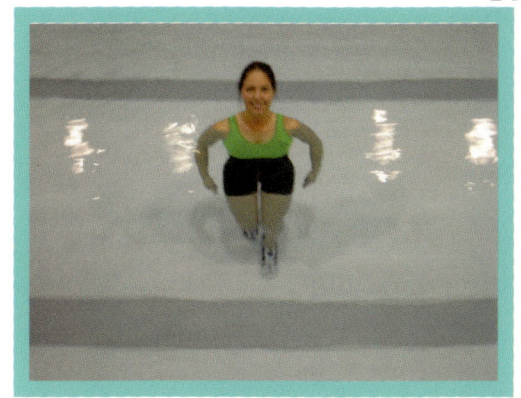

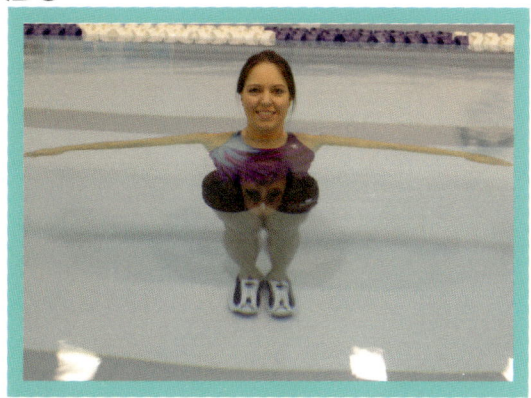

GLOVES

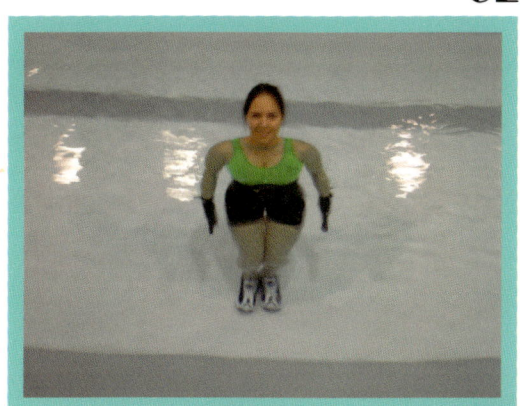

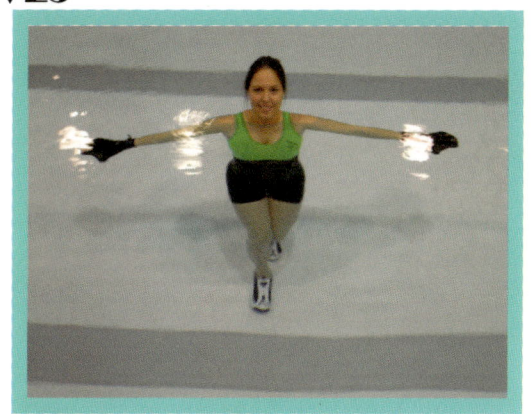

WATER WINGS

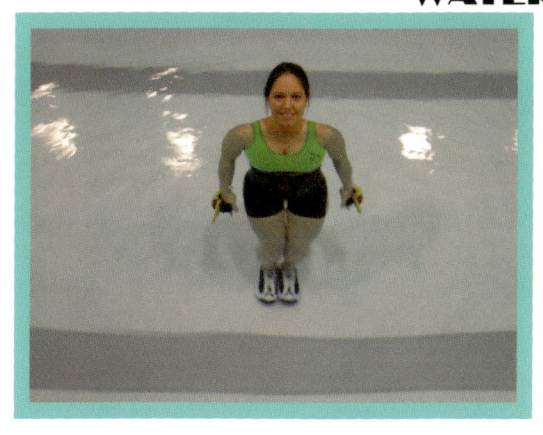

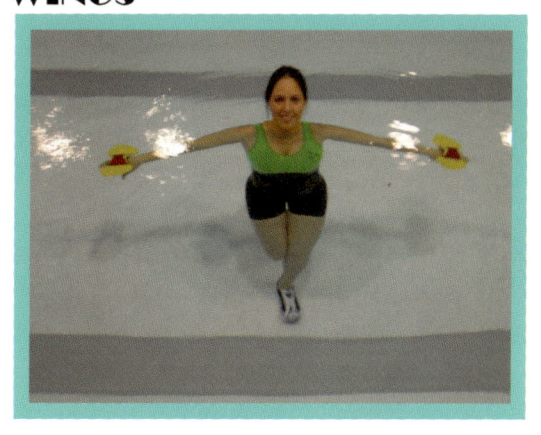

- Stand neutral
- Shoulders underwater
- Hands open to side facing thighs

Raise arms straight out to sides
Continue until hands are level with shoulders
Pull back to start position

✓ Pushing upward will work the middle shoulders (medial deltoids)
✓ Pulling downward creates work for the central back (latissimus dorsi) muscle
✓ Avoid breaking the surface of the water

AQUA TONE

LATERAL RAISES Target Muscle: Medial Deltoid

BANDS

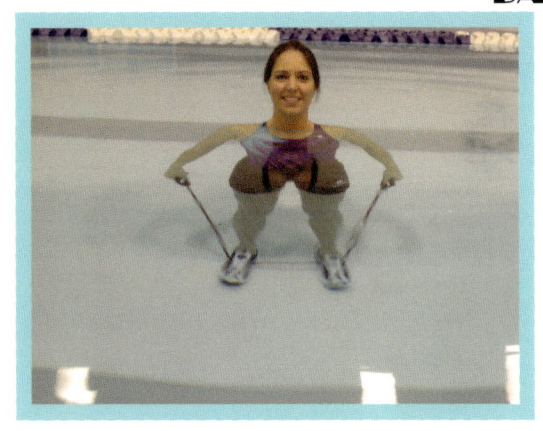

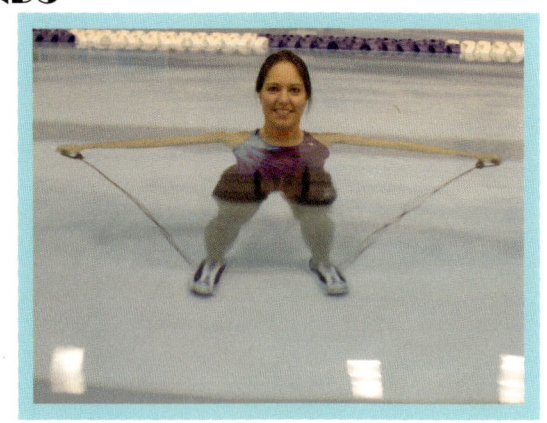

- Stand neutral/shoulders underwater
- Hands holding bands at side
- Bands anchored under feet

Raise bands to shoulder level
Control bands back to starting position

WEIGHTS

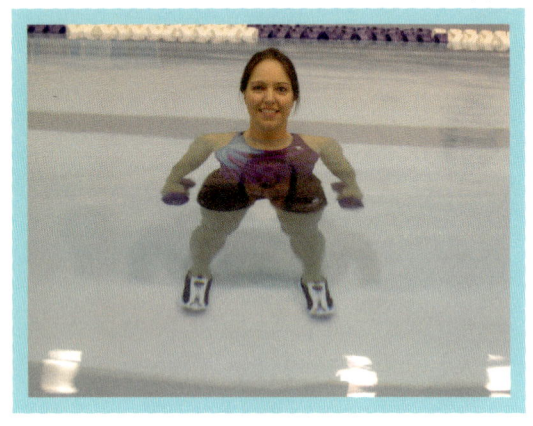

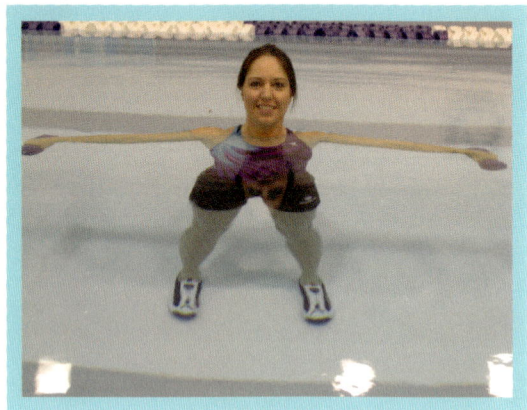

- Stand neutral/shoulders underwater
- Hands holding weights at side

Raise weights level with shoulders
Control weights back to starting position

✓ Feet should stay flat on floor
✓ Keep from shrugging shoulders to assist in raising weights
✓ Avoid breaking the surface of the water

AQUA TONE

FRONT RAISES AND PULL DOWNS Target Muscles: Anterior Deltoids/Lats

HANDS

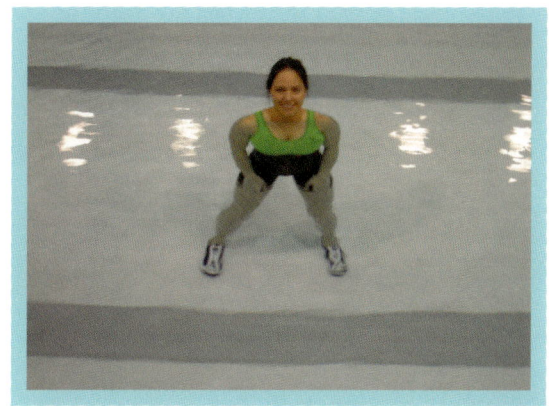

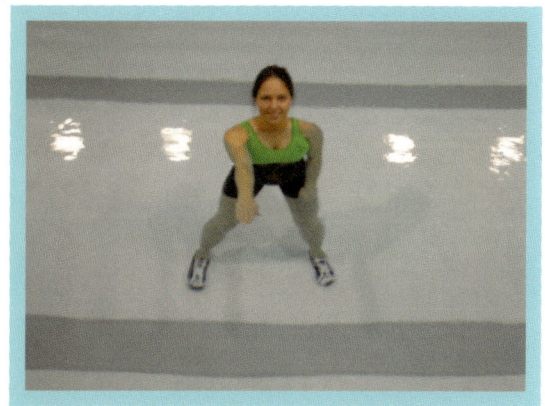

GLOVES

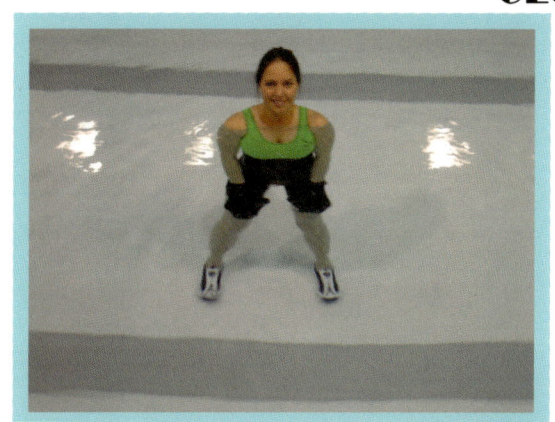

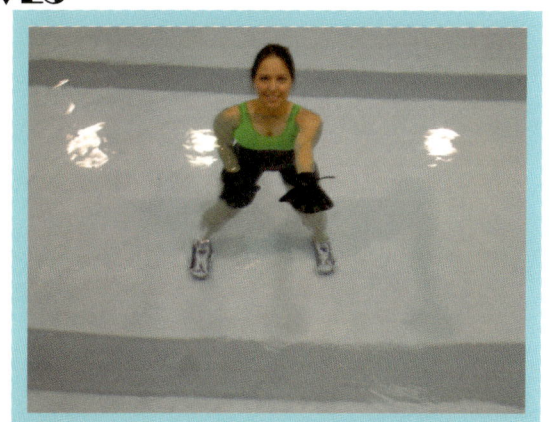

WATER WINGS

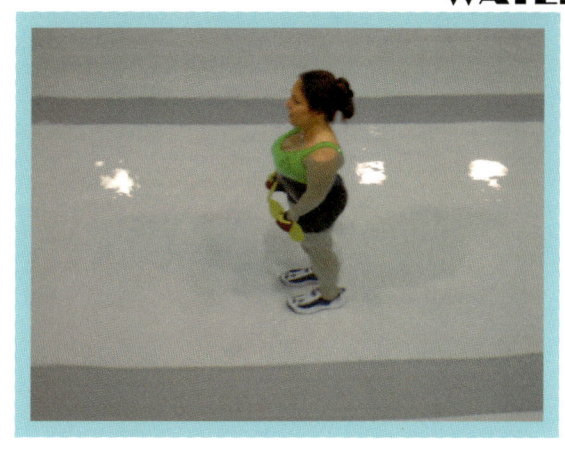

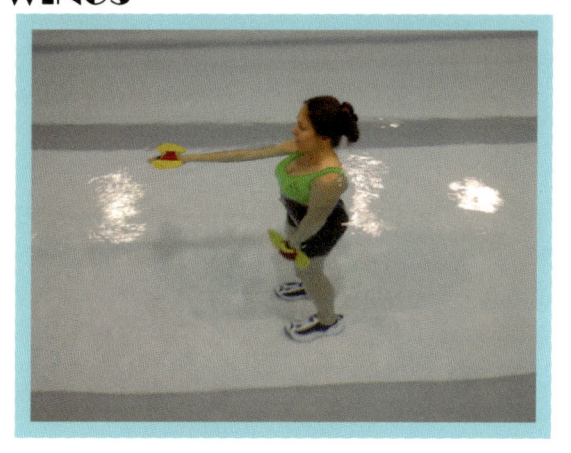

- Stand neutral/Shoulders underwater
- Hands in front of body
- Palms facing body

Raise one arm at a time
Continue until hands are level with shoulders
Pull downward to starting position

✓ **Pushing upward will work the front shoulder (anterior deltoid)**
✓ **Pulling down will create work for the central back (latissimus dorsi) muscle**
✓ **Avoid breaking the surface of the water**

AQUA TONE

FRONT RAISES Target Muscle: Anterior Deltoid

BANDS

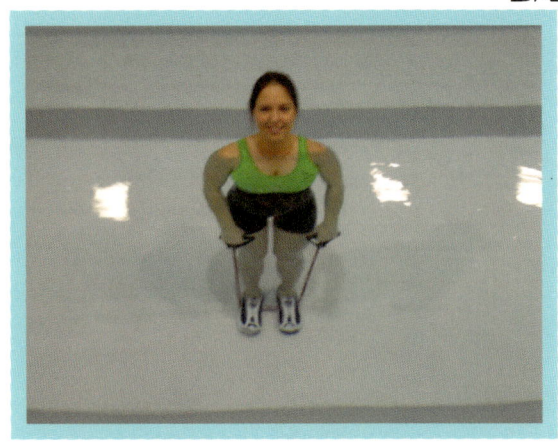

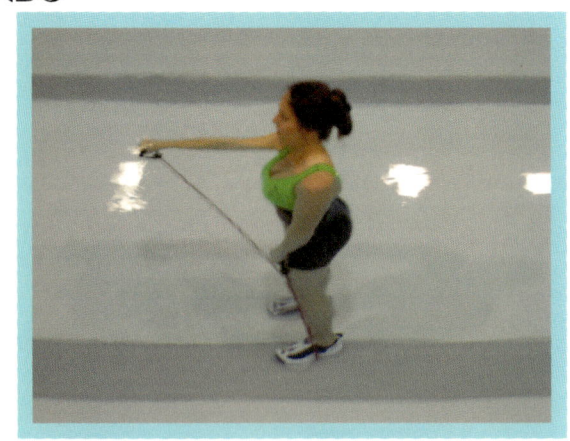

- Stand neutral/shoulders underwater
- Hold bands in front of body
- Palms facing toward body

Raise one arm at a time
Continue until hand is level with shoulder
Control band back to starting position

WEIGHTS

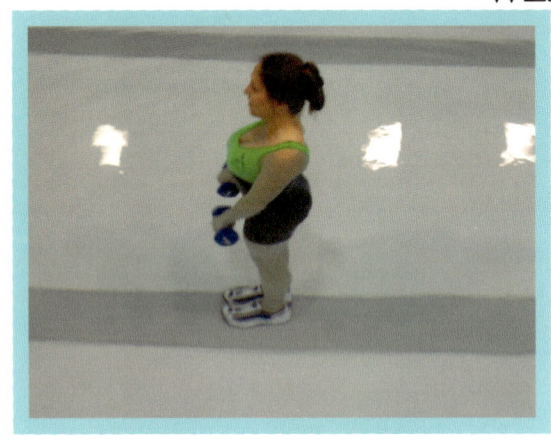

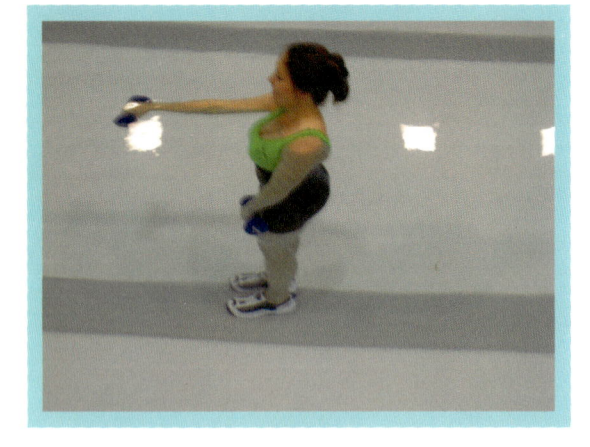

- Stand neutral/shoulders underwater
- Hold weights in front of body
- Palms facing body

Raise one arm at a time
Continue until hand is level with shoulder
Control weight back to starting position

✓ **Avoid breaking the surface of the water**

AQUA TONE

OVERHEAD PRESS Target Muscles: Medial Deltoids/Upper Trapezius

BANDS

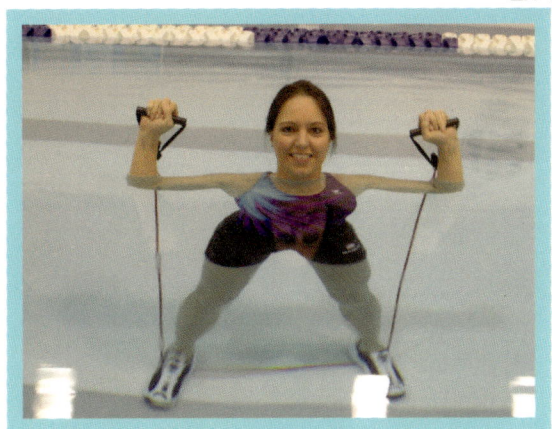

- Stand neutral/shoulders underwater
- Feet hip width apart
- Band anchored under feet
- Forearm and upper arm at 90 degree
- Wrists inline with elbows (neutral)

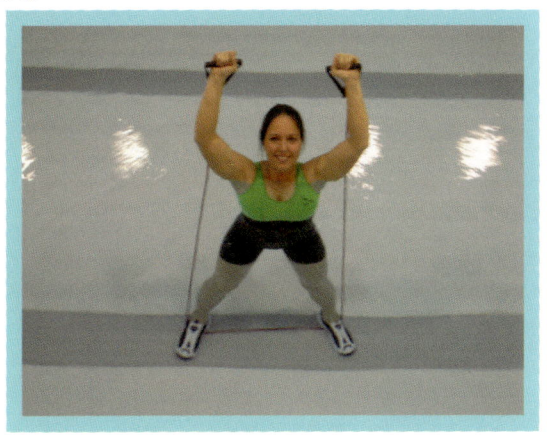

Raise arms above head
Keep wrists neutral
Control bands back to starting position

WEIGHTS

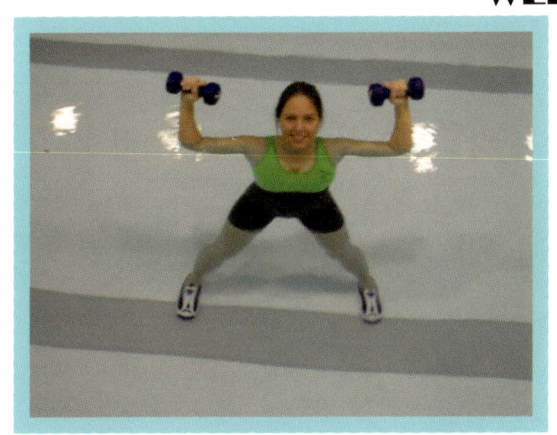

- Stand neutral/Shoulders underwater
- Feet hip width apart
- Hold weights/palms facing forward
- Forearm and upper arm at 90 degree
- Wrists inline with elbows (neutral)

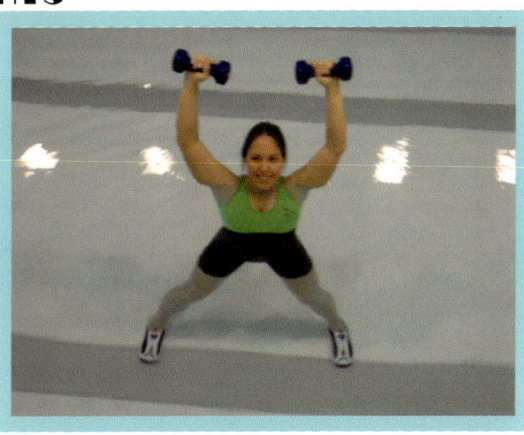

Raise arms above head
Keep wrists neutral
Control weights back to starting position

AQUA TONE

BICEP CURLS Target Muscle: Bicep brachii

HANDS

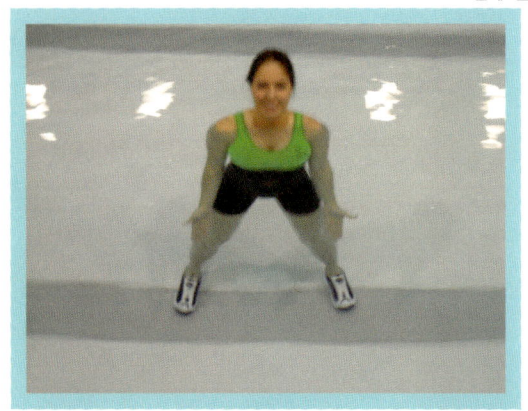

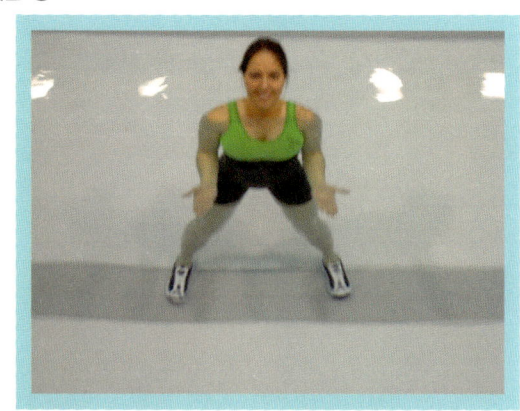

GLOVES

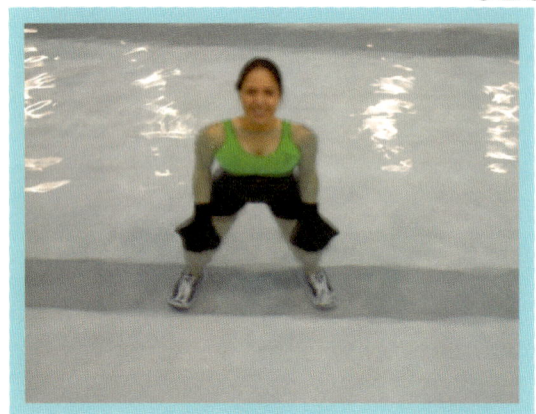

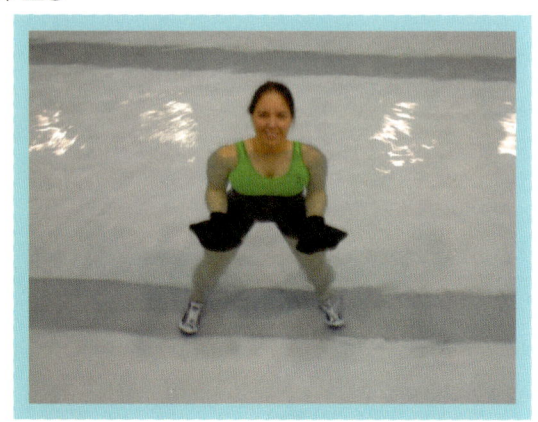

WATER WINGS

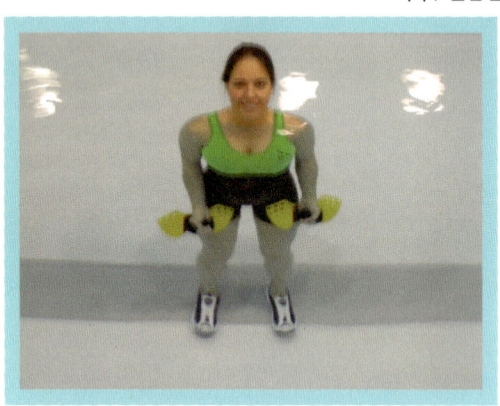

- Stand neutral/elbows close to side
- Hand open/facing up/fingers together
- Hand/wrist/forearm in line with shoulder
- Elbow slightly bent at thighs

Pull hands up towards shoulders
Pull to surface (not out of water)
Keep wrists locked in neutral (don't curl)
Turn hands/Slice back to starting position

✓ **Keep elbows close to body and aligned with shoulder when pulling hands towards shoulders**

AQUA TONE

BICEP CURLS Target Muscle: Bicep brachii

BANDS

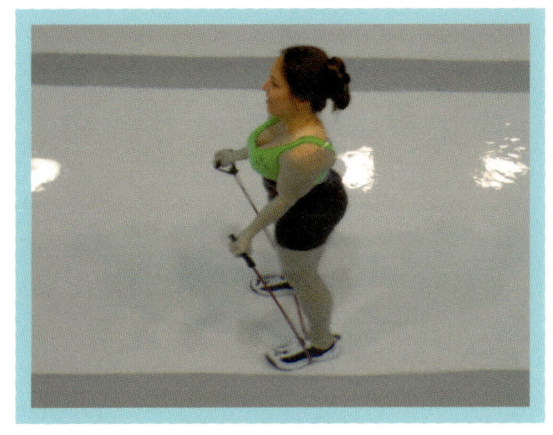

- Stand neutral/elbows close to side
- Hand/wrist/forearm in line with shoulder
- Band anchored under both feet
- Hands on thighs/elbow slightly bent

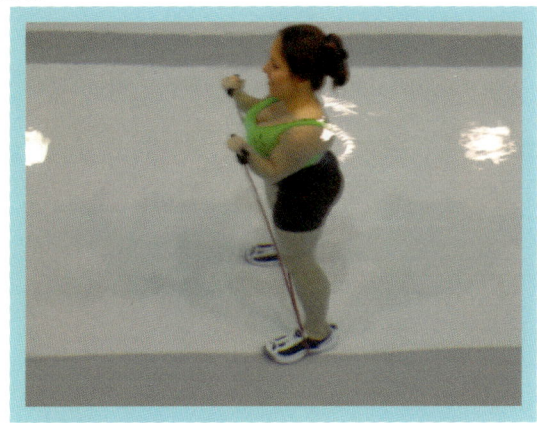

Pull hands upward toward shoulders
Stay in line with shoulders
Keep wrists locked in neutral (don't curl)
Pull to surface (not out of water)
Control bands back to starting position

FOAM BARBELLS

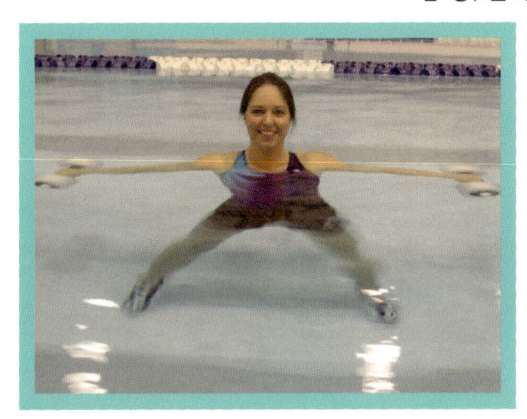

- Stand neutral
- Hold barbells out to both sides of body
- Arms/hands/wrists in line with shoulders

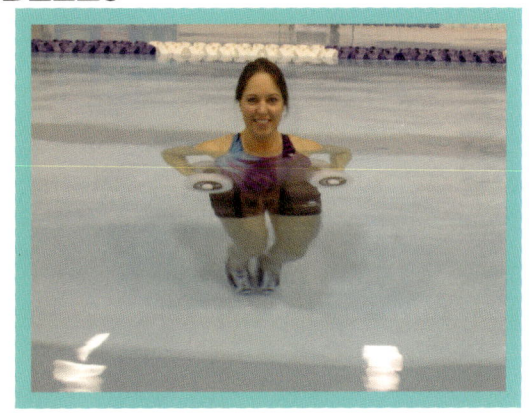

Bend elbows/pull barbells downward
Pull to waist
Control barbells back to starting position

This is easier when performed with a jumping jack motion

AQUA TONE

BICEP CURLS Target Muscle: Biceps brachii

WEIGHTS

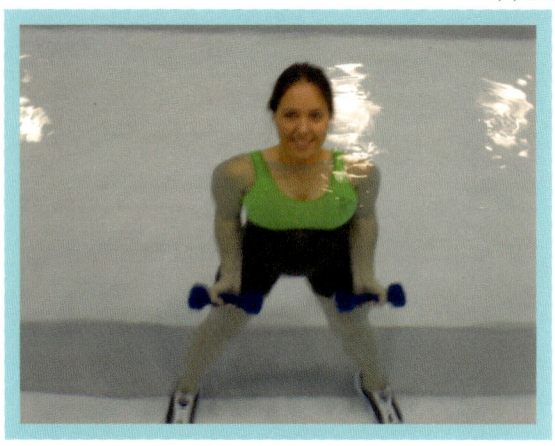

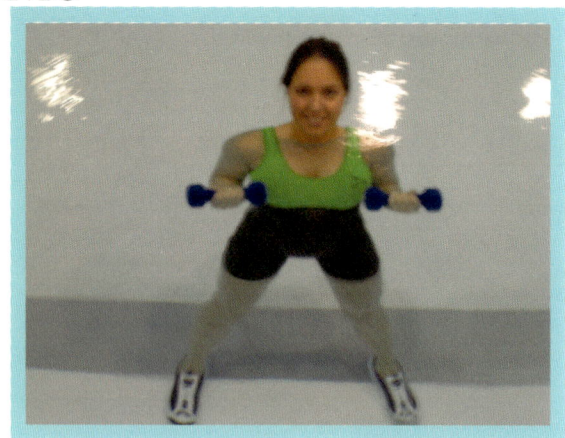

- Stand neutral/elbows close to side
- Palms facing up
- Hands/wrists/forearm in line with shoulders
- Elbows slightly bent/resting on thighs

Pull weight to surface bending the elbows
Wrists locked in neutral (don't curl)
Hands/wrists/forearm in line with shoulders
Control weight back to starting position

✓ **Keep elbows close to body and aligned with shoulder when pulling hands toward shoulders**

HAMMER CURLS Target Muscles: Brachioradialis/Bracialis

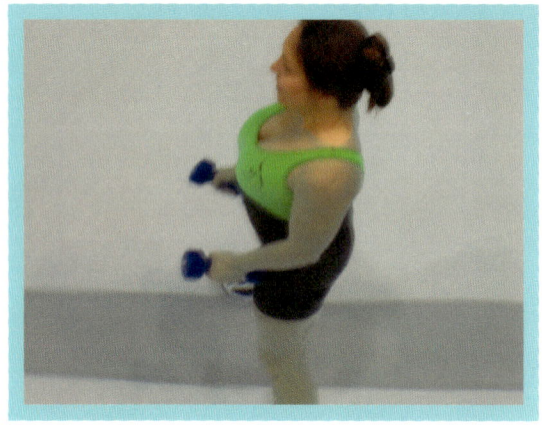

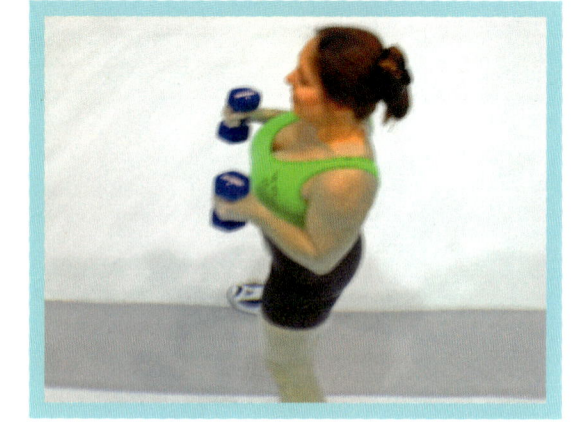

- Stand neutral/elbows close to side
- Hold weights in vertical position
- Hands/wrists/forearms in line with shoulders

Pull weight to surface (not out of water)
Keep elbows close to side
Control weight to starting position

This can also be performed with one arm at a time

HAMMER CURLS KEEP SHOULDERS IN NEUTRAL AND MAY BE EASIER ON SHOULDERS THAN BICEP CURLS IF INJURY CONDITIONS EXIST.

AQUA TONE

BICEP CURL/HAMMER CURL COMBINATION WITH WEIGHTS

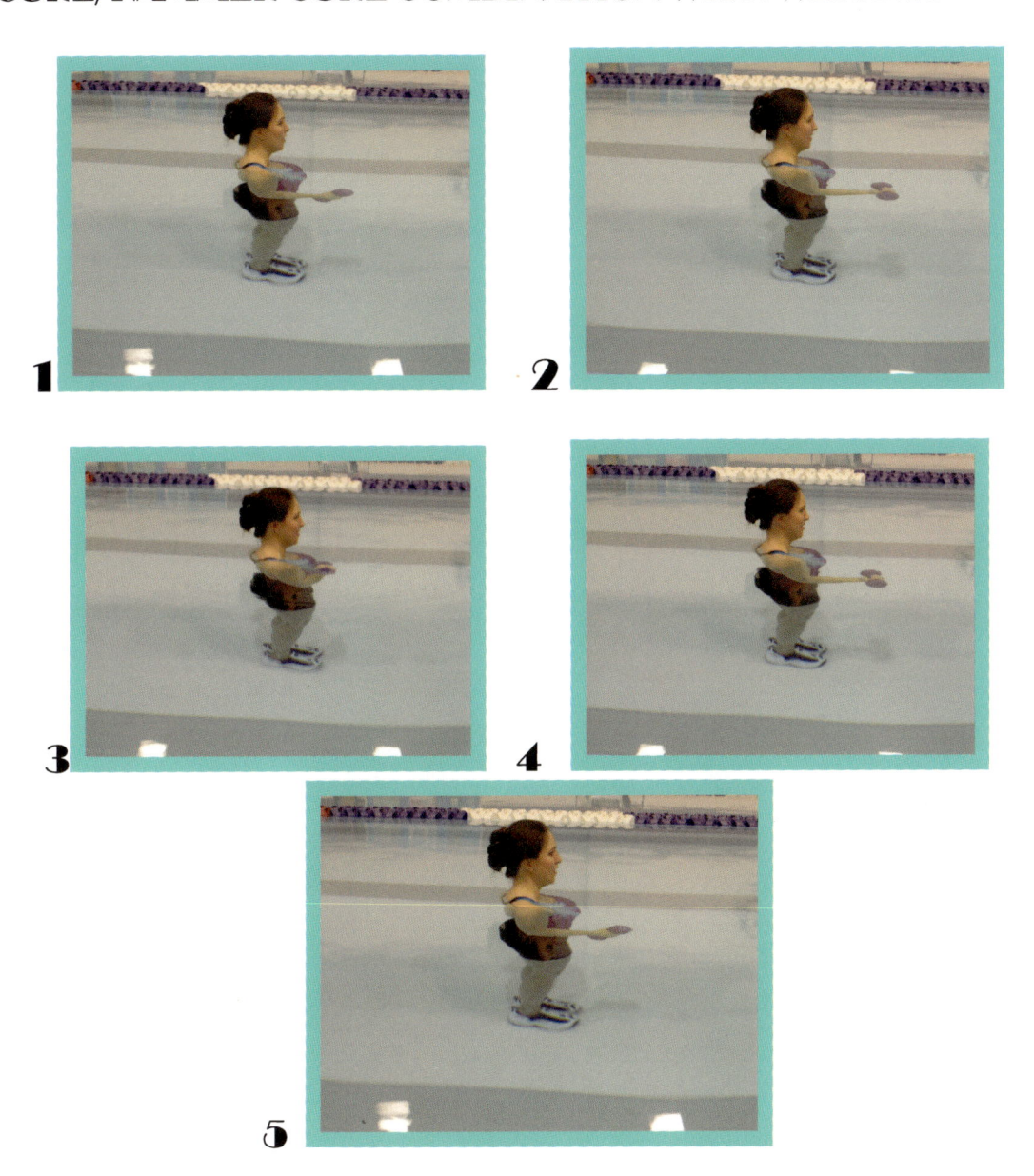

1. Stand neutral/ Begin with hammer curl
2. Turn wrist and forearm to bicep curl when upper and lower arm are at 90 degree angle
3. Complete bicep curl
4. Return to 90 degree angle with bicep curl
5. Turn wrist and forearm/completing with hammer curl

AQUA TONE

PUSHDOWNS Target Muscle: Triceps

HANDS

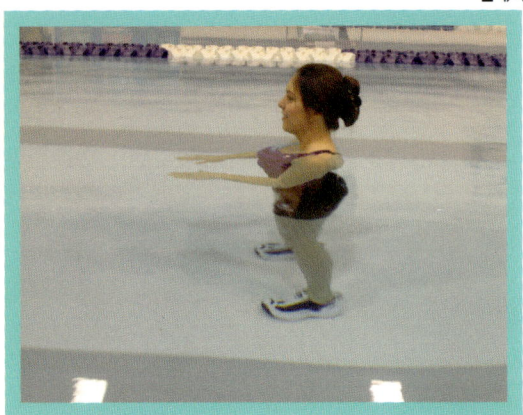

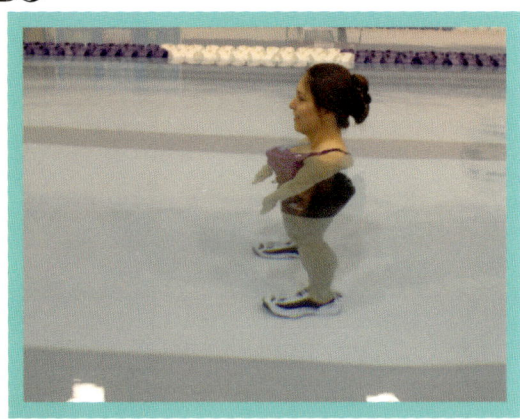

GLOVES

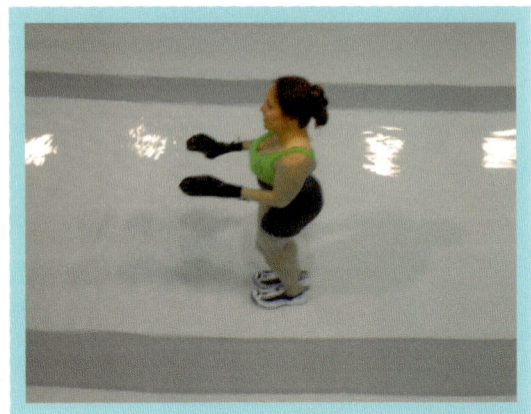

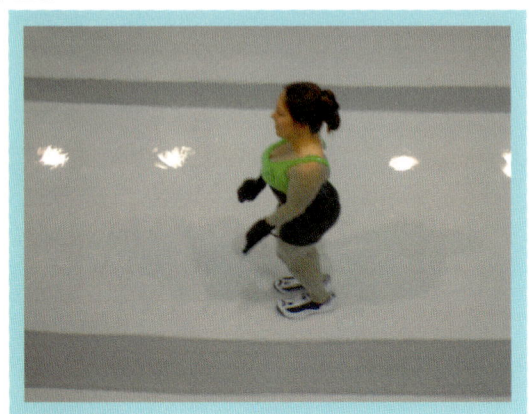

WATER WINGS

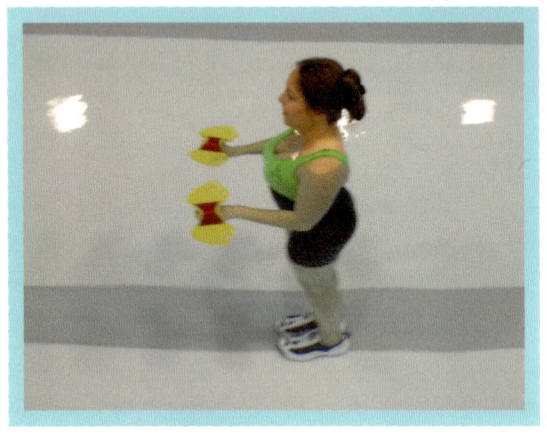

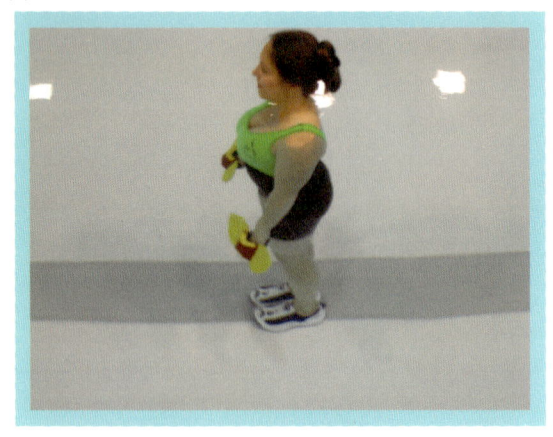

- Stand neutral/triceps underwater
- Palms facing down
- Elbows close to sides
- Hands in line with shoulders

Press downward to thighs
Keep elbows close to side
Turn palms inward and slice back to start

These can be combined with bicep curls simply by rotating the hands (palms up) at the end of the pushdown and performing the bicep curl as directed

AQUA TONE

PUSHDOWNS Target Muscle: Triceps

NOODLE

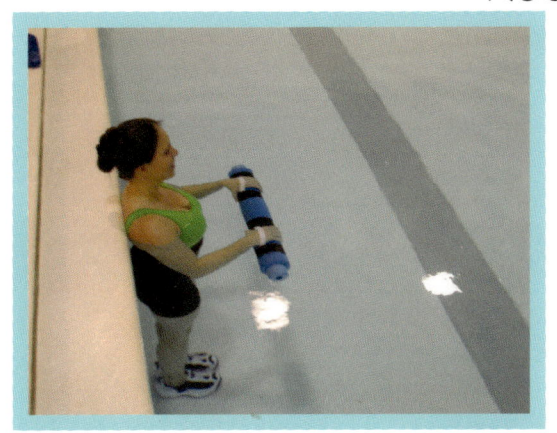

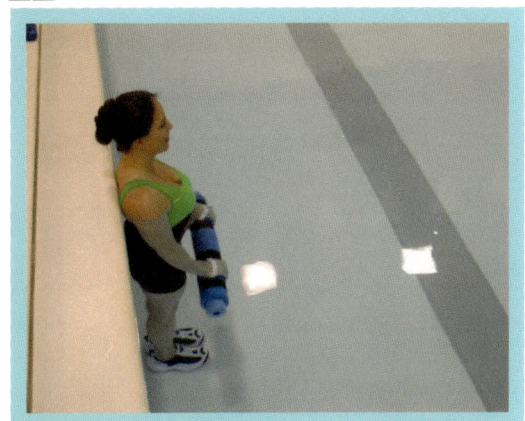

SWIM BARBELL

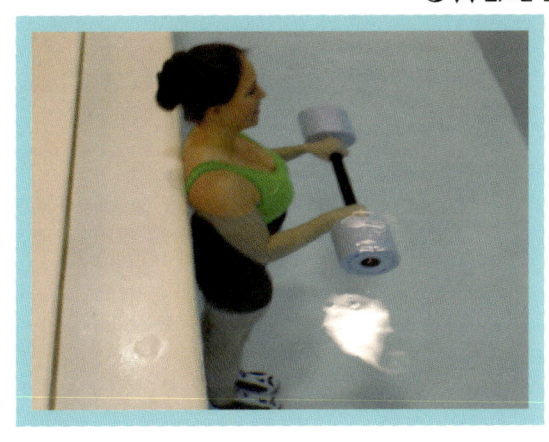

- Stand neutral/Elbows close to sides
- Hands in line with shoulders
- Equipment just under surface of water

Press down with hands (from the elbows)
Keep elbows close to sides
Return to start

✓ **Avoid breaking the surface of the water**

NOODLE ALLOWS FOR A NON-GRIPPING HAND POSITION FOR THOSE WITH ARTHRITIS OR CARPAL TUNNEL (SEE ADAPTED NOODLE SECTION)

AQUA TONE

DIPS Target Muscle: Triceps

HANDS

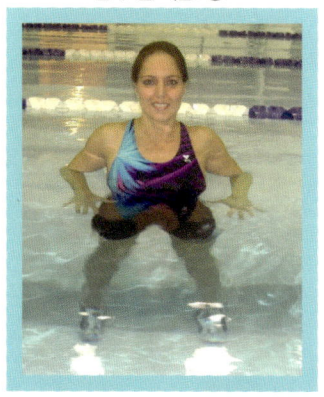

GLOVES

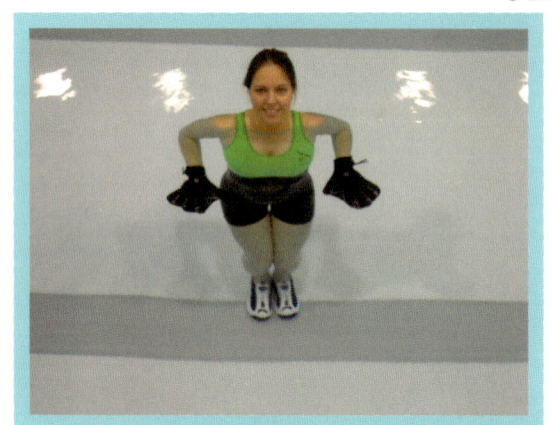

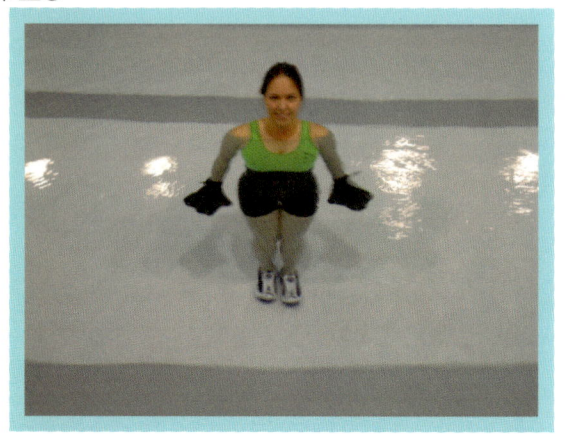

FOAM BARBELLS

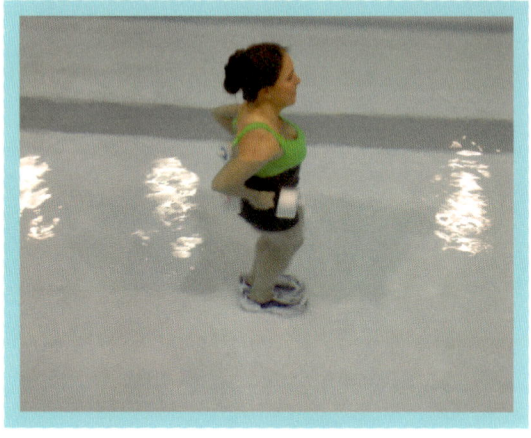

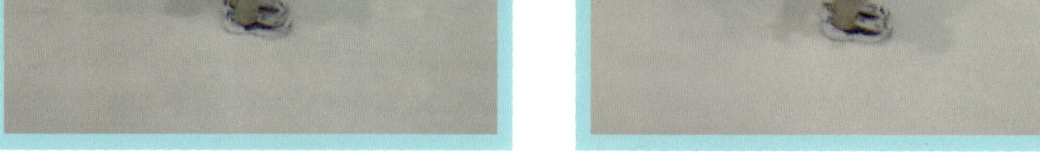

- **Stand neutral/hands at hips**
- **Elbows are close to and behind body**

Press down
Keep elbows slightly bent/Do not lock
Return to start

AQUA TONE

RUNNING CHEST PRESS Target Muscle: Pectoralis Major

HANDS

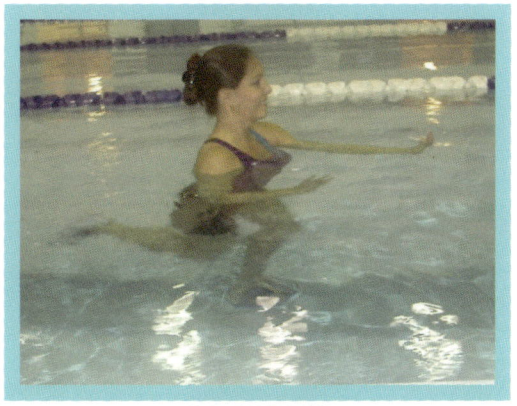

GLOVES

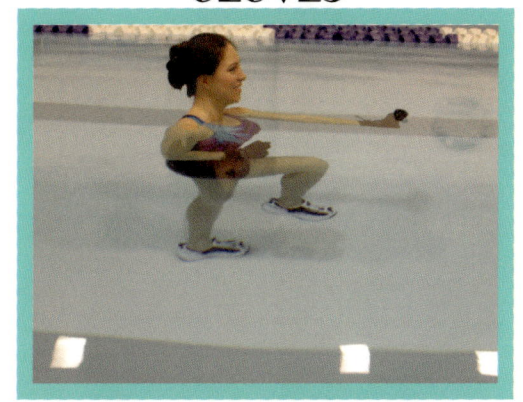

FOAM BARBELLS

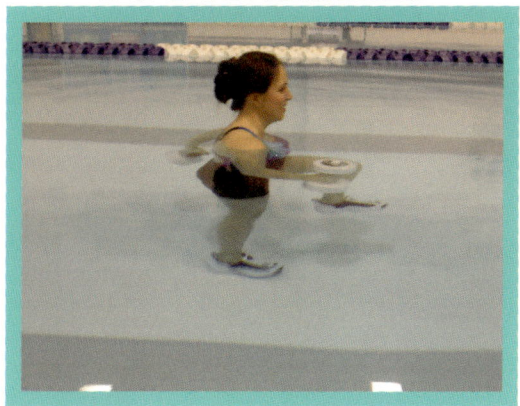

- Running in neutral position
- Alternate Arms in jogging motion
- Keep open hands or equipment under surface of water
- Keep elbows close to body
- Elbows should stay slightly bent on the pressing motion

AQUA TONE

CHEST PRESS Target Muscle: Pectoralis Major

BANDS

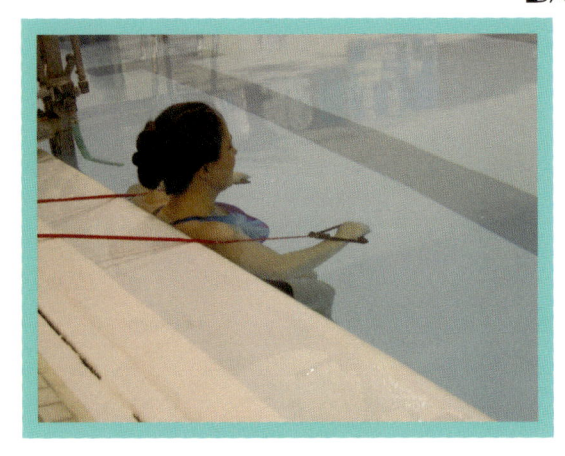

- Chest under water
- Shoulders/Elbow at 90 degree
- Wrists neutral
- Palms facing downward

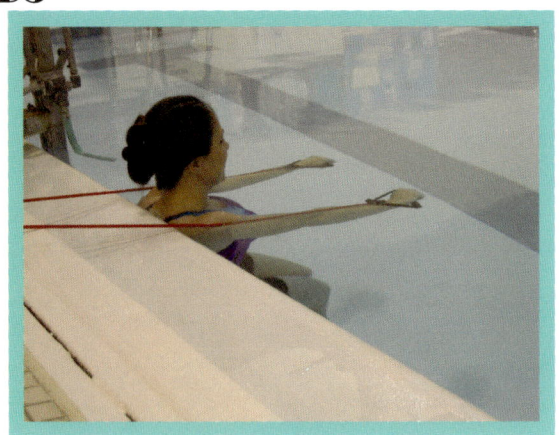

Press outward
Keep elbows slightly bent/Don't lock
Return to start

ALTERNATE CHEST PRESS

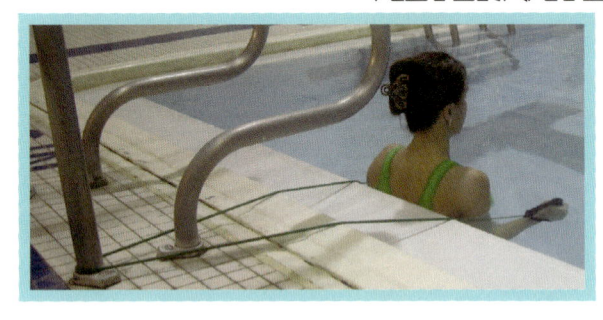

- Elbows are low and next to body
- Palms are facing inward

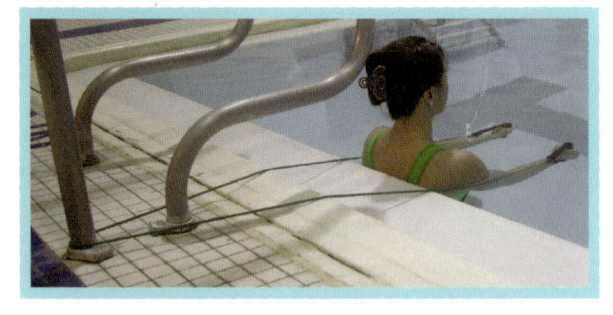

Press outward keeping elbows slightly bent
Return to start

ALTERNATE CHEST PRESS KEEPS SHOULDERS IN NEUTRAL AND CAN POSSIBLY BE USED INSTEAD OF REGULAR CHEST PRESS IF SHOULDER CONDITIONS OR INJURIES EXIST.

AQUA TONE

FLYS Target Muscles: Pectoralis Major/Deltoids/Trapezius

HANDS

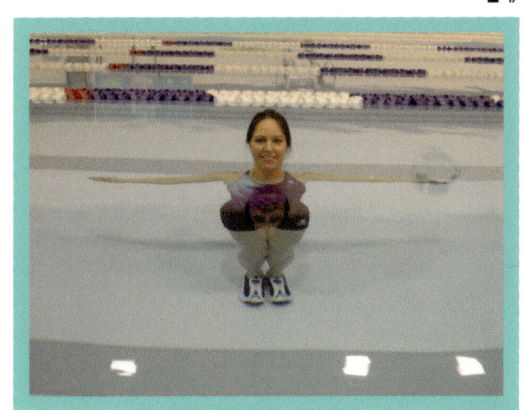

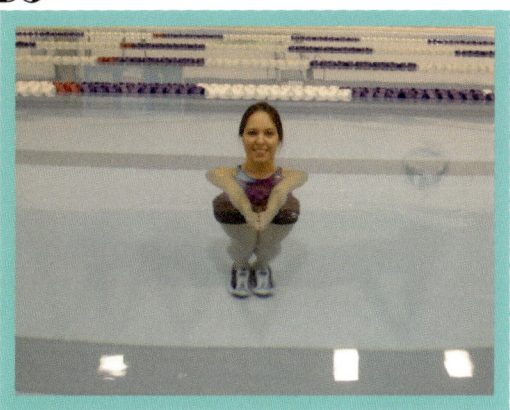

GLOVES

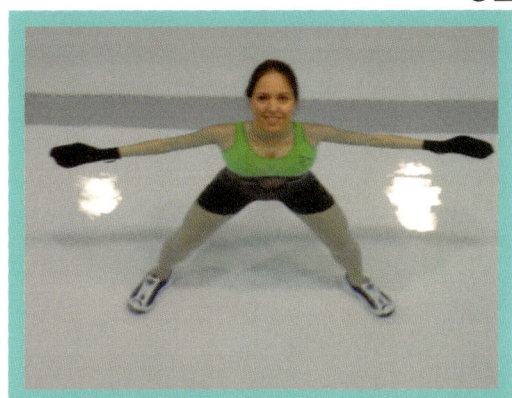

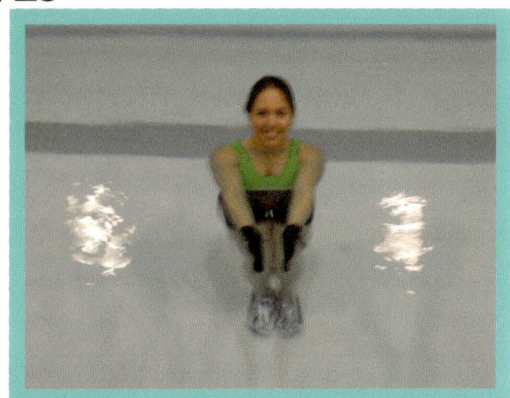

BARBELLS

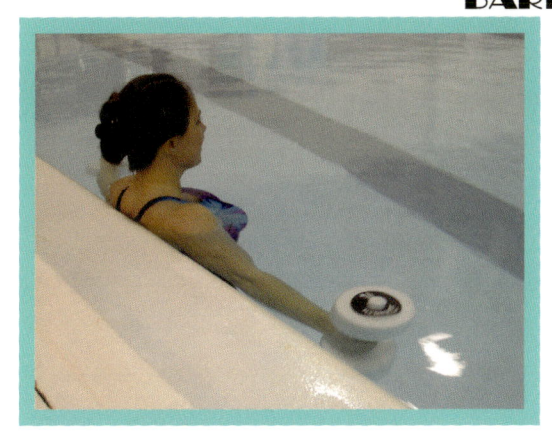

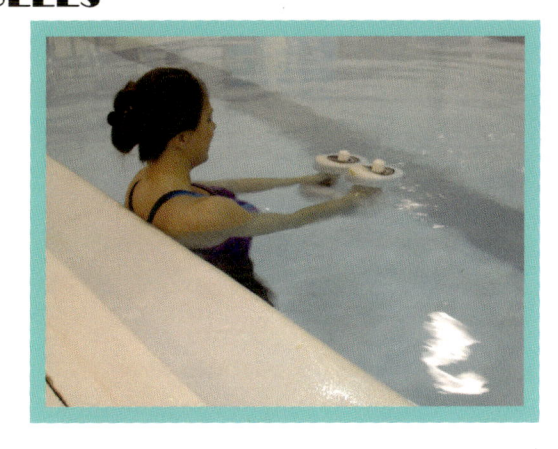

- Stand neutral/Arms extended out
- Hands are open/Palms facing forward

Pull hands/barbells toward each other
Push forcefully back to start
Squeeze shoulder blades together

✓ **Pulling inward works the chest (pectoralis major) and the front shoulders (anterior deltoids)**
✓ **Pushing back to start creates work for the rear shoulders (posterior deltoids) and the upper back (trapezius).**

AQUA TONE

COMPOUND ROW Target Muscles: Latissimus Dorsi/Posterior Deltoids

BANDS

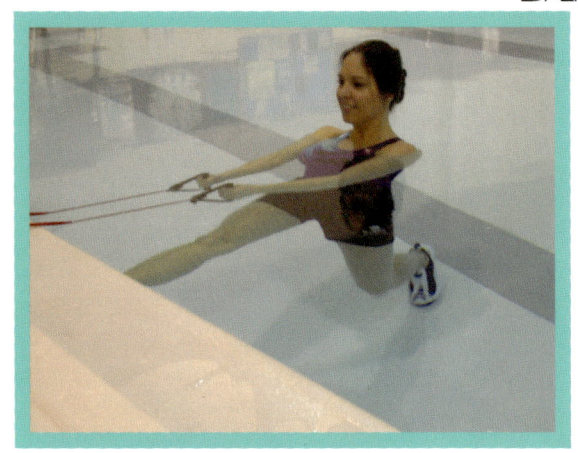

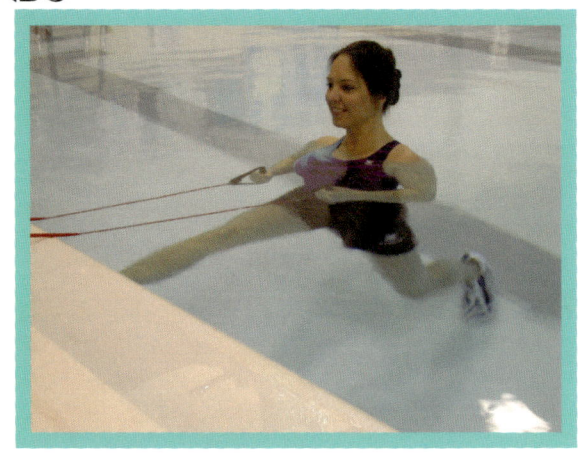

- Stand neutral/back under water
- Hold bands/Palms facing each other
- Placing foot on wall gives balance

Slowly pull back /squeeze shoulder blades
Elbows stay low and close to body
Control bands on return

This hand position keeps shoulders in neutral

✓ Do not allow bands to pull shoulders forward on the return
✓ Avoid rocking motion
✓ Keep elbows slightly bent on the start and the return

COMPOUND ROW (ALTERNATE ARM POSITION)

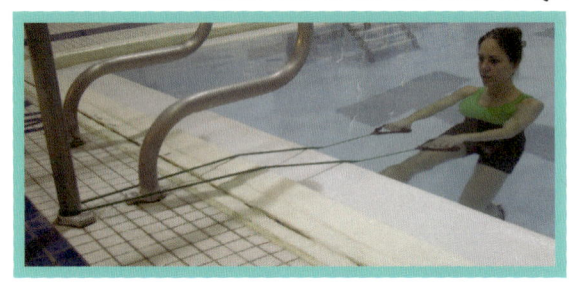

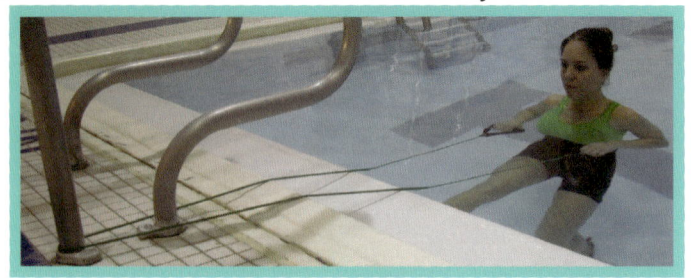

- Use an overhand grip with palms facing downward

Pull back/Squeeze shoulder blades

This hand position involves the trapezius to a greater extent

AQUA TONE

PULLDOWNS Target Muscle: Latissimus Dorsi

BAR

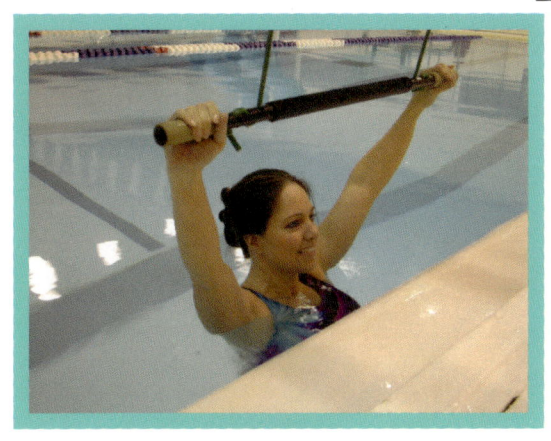

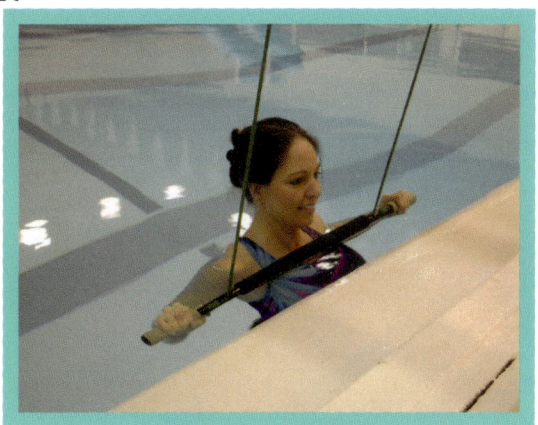

- Stand neutral/facing bar
- Grip is overhand and wide
- Elbows slightly bent

Pull bar down to upper chest
Arch back slightly/bring elbows back
Return to start

✓ **Do not allow bands to pull shoulders upward when returning back to start**
✓ **Keep head over shoulders in neutral when arching back**
✓ **Avoid leaning back**

SHOULDER SHRUGS Target Muscle: Trapezius

WEIGHTS

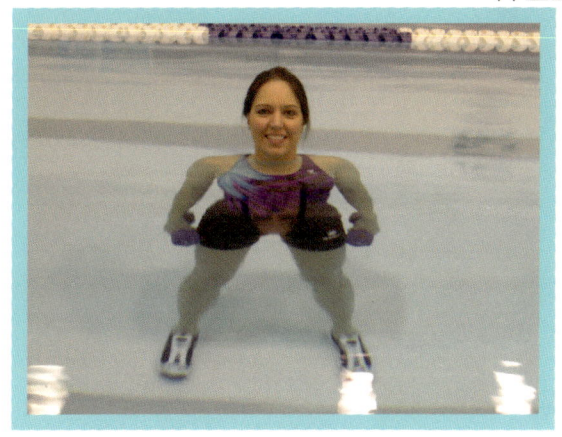

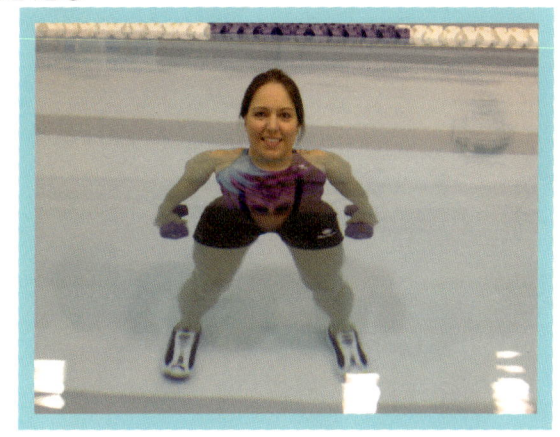

- Stand neutral/arms at sides
- Shoulders underwater

Shrug shoulders as high as possible
Return to start

Beginners can start without weights

AQUA TONE

HIP ABDUCTION/ADDUCTION Target Muscles: Gluteus medius/Maximus
Adductor Magnus

LEGS

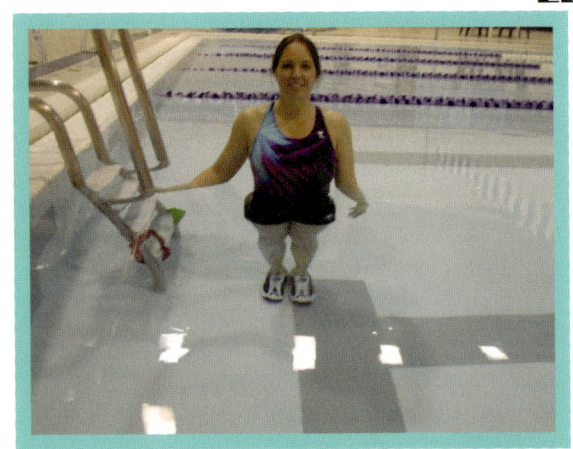

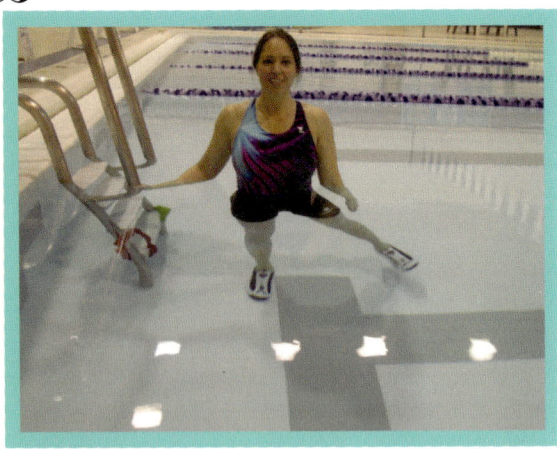

WATER WINGS

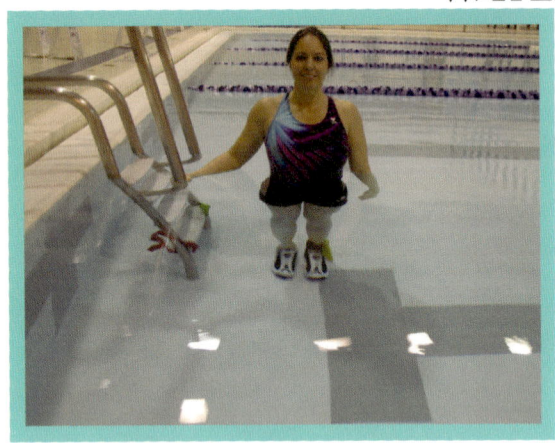

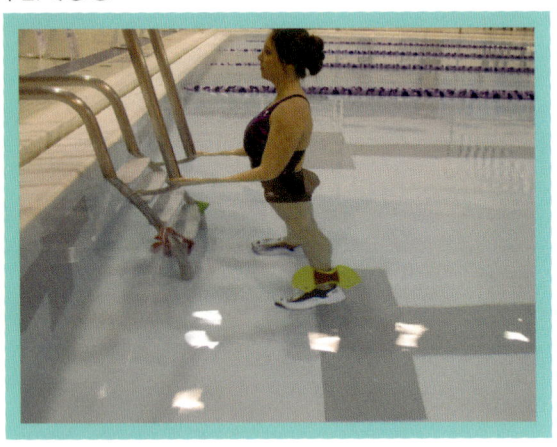

- **Stand neutral/feet together**   **Push outward/pull inward**

  ✓ **Avoid leaning in the opposite direction on the pushing phase**
  ✓ **Keep hip in line with shoulders**

  Range of motion is dependent on individual flexibility

AQUA TONE

HIP ABDUCTION Target Muscles: Gluteus Medius/Maximus

ANCHORED LATEX BAND

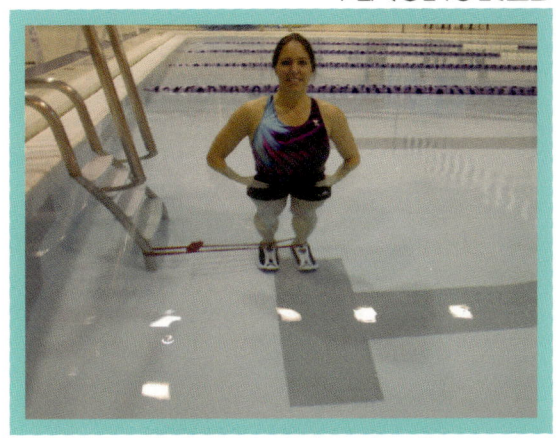

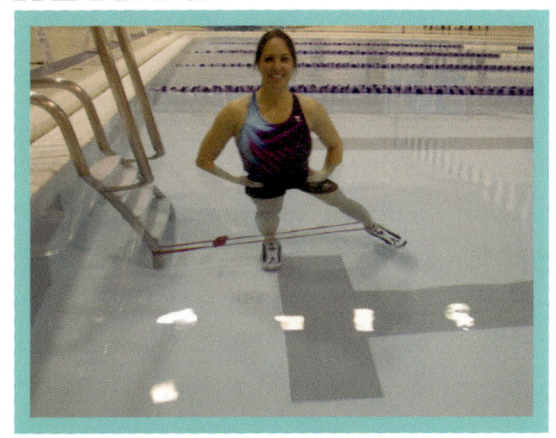

SELF ANCHORED RUBBER BUTTERFLY BAND

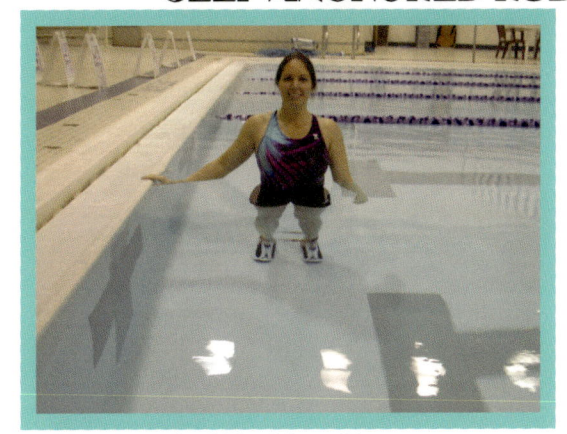

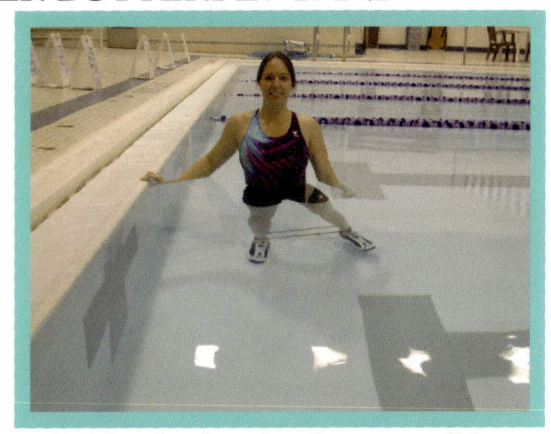

- **Stand neutral/feet together** **Pull band outward as far as possible**

ANKLE WEIGHT

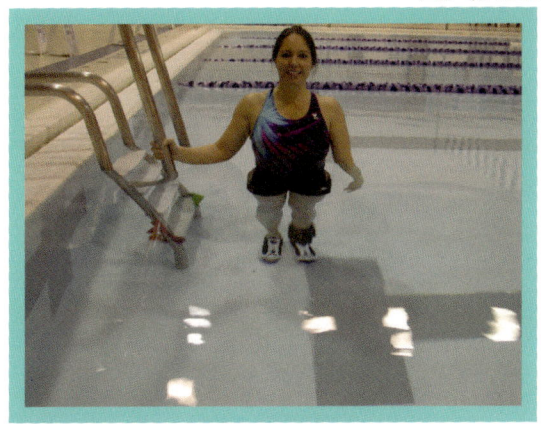

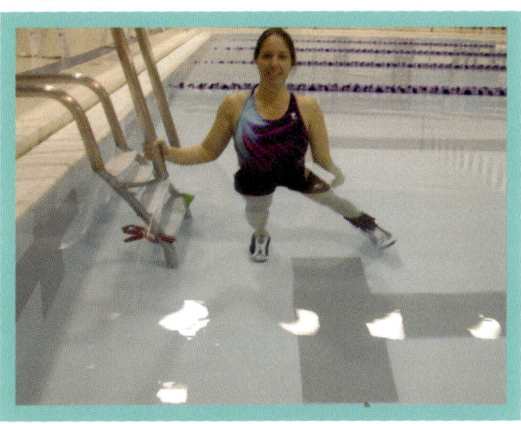

- **Stand neutral/feet together** **Push weight outward as far as possible**

✓ **Avoid leaning in the opposite direction on the pulling (bands) or pushing (ankle weights) phase**
Range of motion is dependent on individual flexibility

AQUA TONE

LEG ADDUCTION Target Muscles: Adductors

ANCHORED BAND

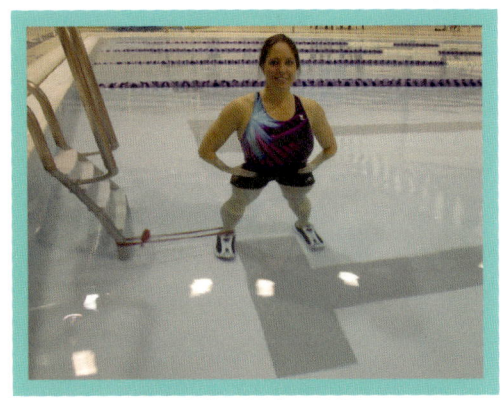

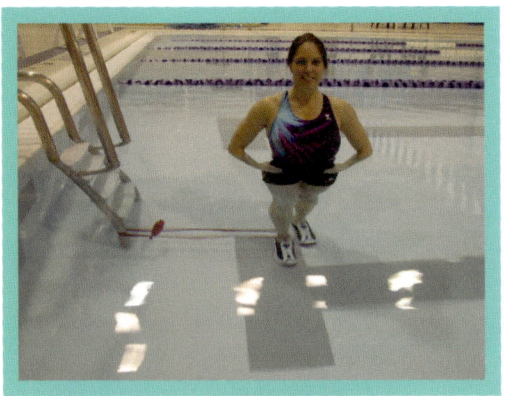

- **Stand neutral/feet hip width apart** **Pull band toward midline**

Resistance can be adjusted by distance from anchor and length of band as well as color of band
DO NOT CROSS MIDLINE IF HIP REPLACEMENT EXISTS

BOUYANCY CUFFS

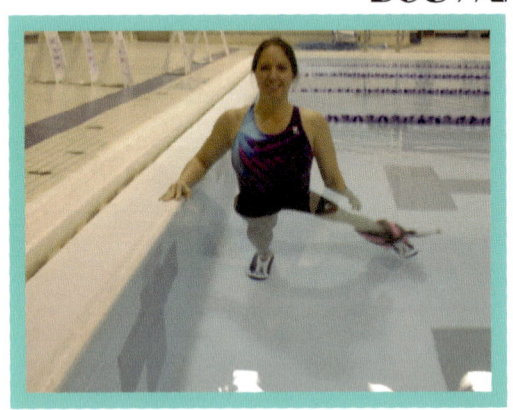

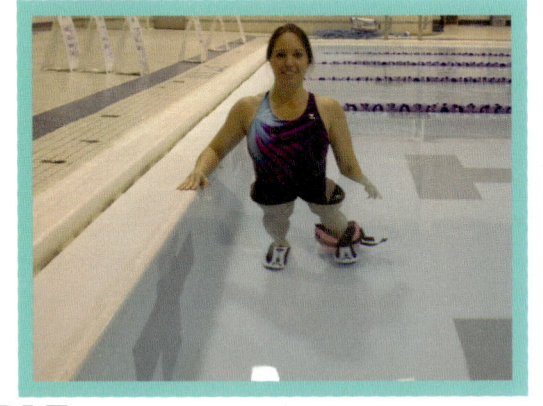

NOODLE

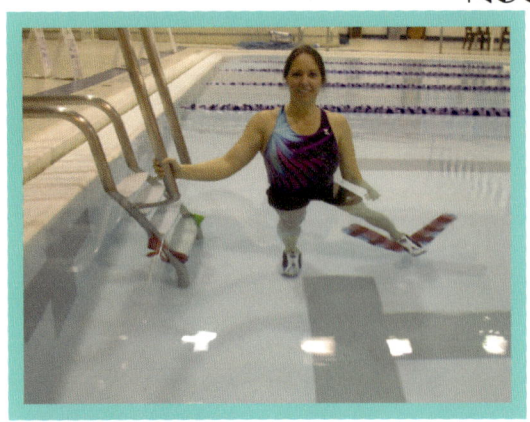

- **Stand neutral** **Pull leg toward midline**
- **Control leg as it extends away from midline**
- **Keep hips in neutral**

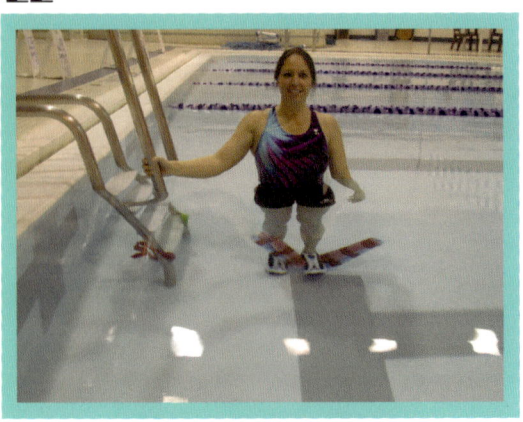

AQUA TONE

STRAIGHT LEG KICK BACKS Target Muscle: Gluteus Maximus

LEGS

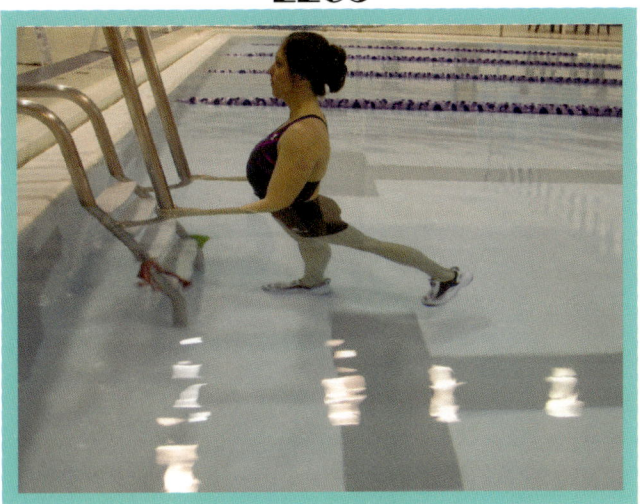

WATER WINGS

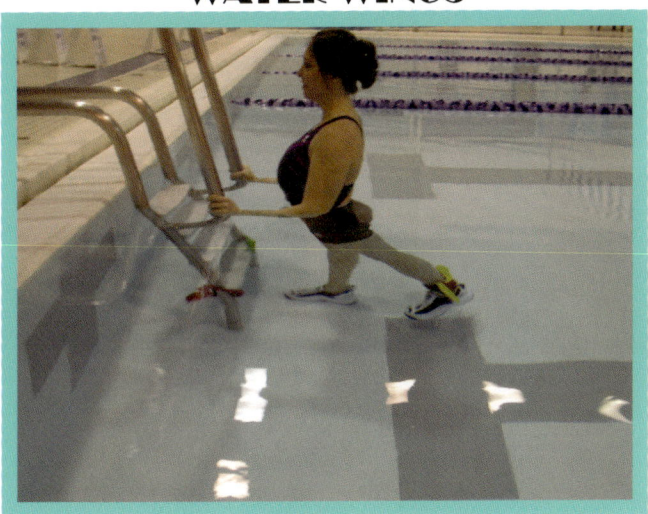

- **Stand neutral/feet together**
- **Tighten glutes**
- **Push leg back**
- **Pull leg back to start**

✓ **Avoid rocking upper torso forward**
✓ **Keep back straight**
✓ **Push from the glutes**

AQUA TONE

STRAIGHT LEG KICK BACK Target Muscle: Gluteus Maximus

ANCHORED BAND

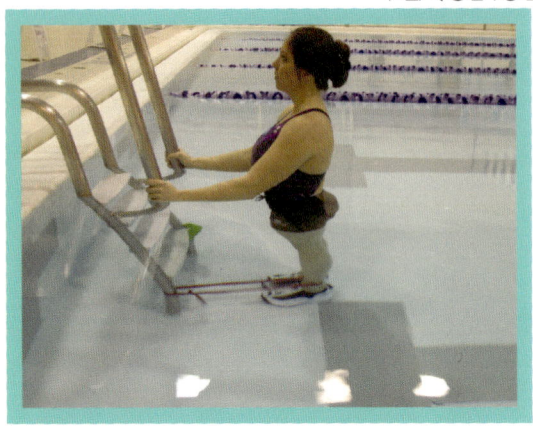

- Stand neutral/feet together
- Tighten glutes

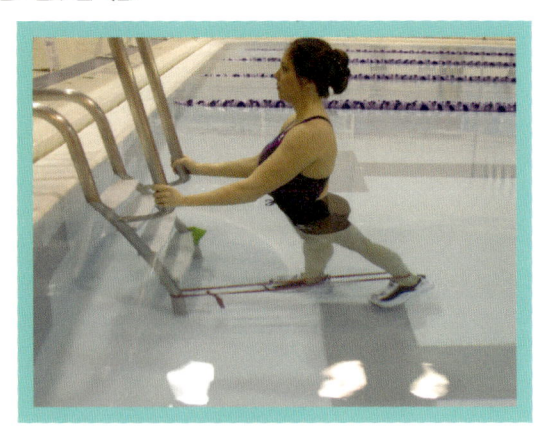

Pull band back
Return to start

ANKLE WEIGHT

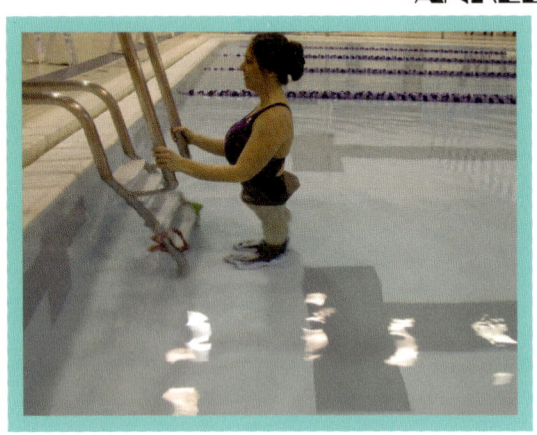

- Stand neutral/feet together
- Tighten glutes

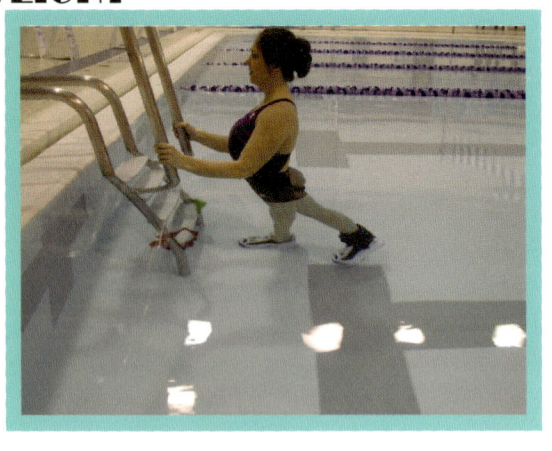

Push leg back
Return to start

✓ Avoid rocking upper torso forward
✓ Keep back straight
✓ Pull or push from the glutes

AQUA TONE

LEG CURL/EXTENSION Target Muscles: Hamstrings/Quadriceps

LEGS

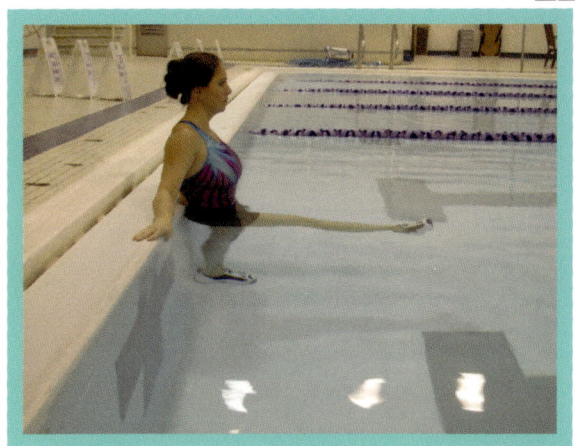

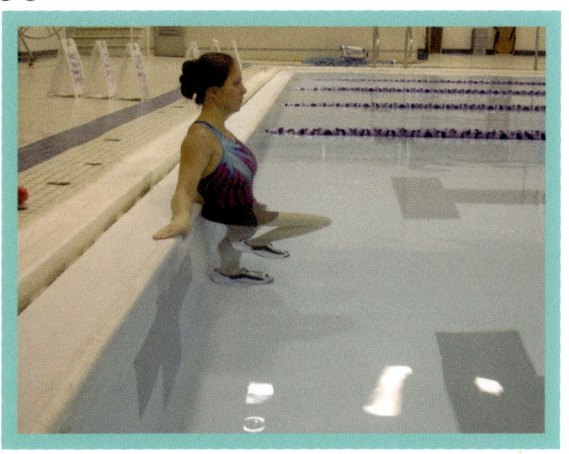

WATER WINGS

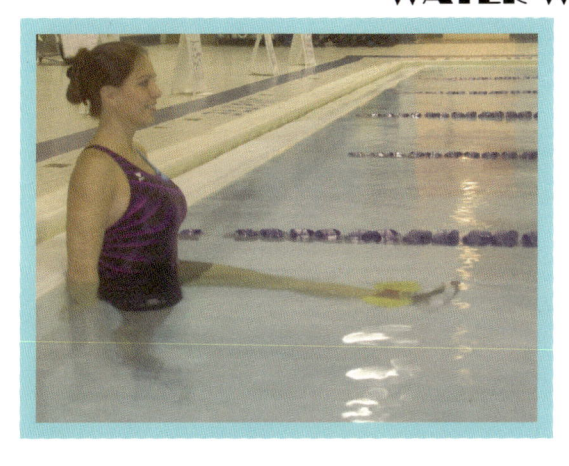

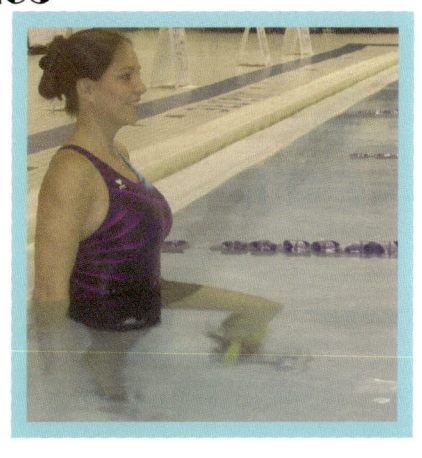

- Stand neutral/leg extended
- Keep knee stationary at hip level
- Keep standing leg slightly bent at the knee

✓ Pulling leg back works the hamstring muscle
✓ Pushing leg back out creates work for the quadricep muscle

Pull lower leg back toward body (flex foot)
Push lower leg back out to extended position

AQUA TONE

LEG CURL Target Muscle : Hamstrings

NOODLE

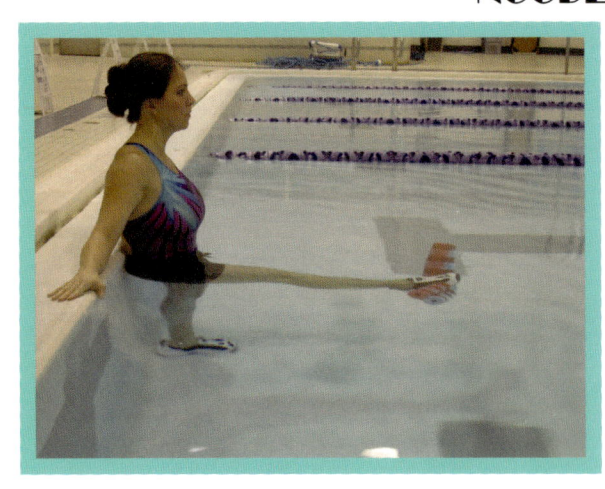

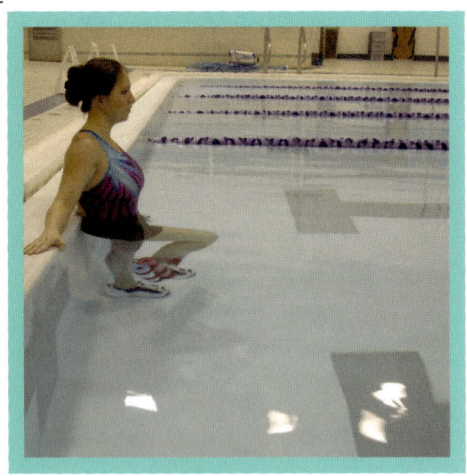

- Stand neutral/place foot on top of noodle
- Extend leg
- Knee stays stationary at hip level

Pull noodle back toward body as far as possible
Control noodle back to extended position

ANKLE WEIGHT

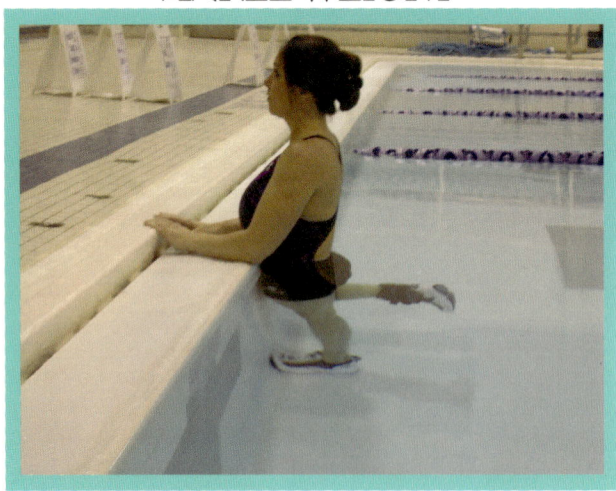

- Stand with feet together in neutral position
- Raise leg toward buttocks
- Return to start

AQUA TONE

QUAD PUSHDOWN/EXTENSION Target Muscle: Quadriceps

NOODLES

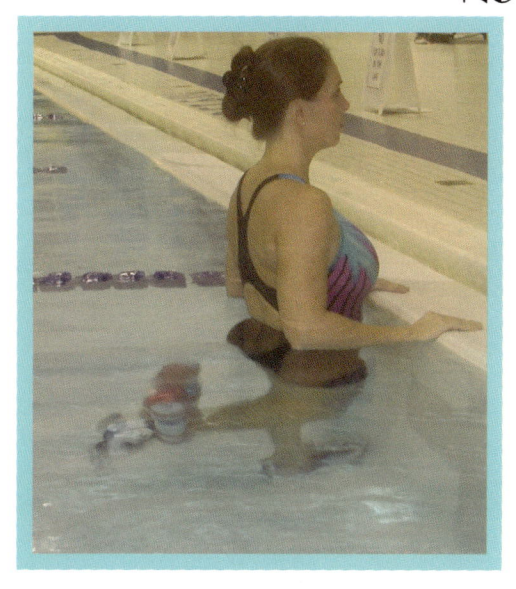

- Stand neutral
- Place top of foot on top of noodle
- Knee is bent with foot in line with knee

Press noodle downward as far as possible
Keep knee stationary
Return to start

ANKLE WEIGHTS

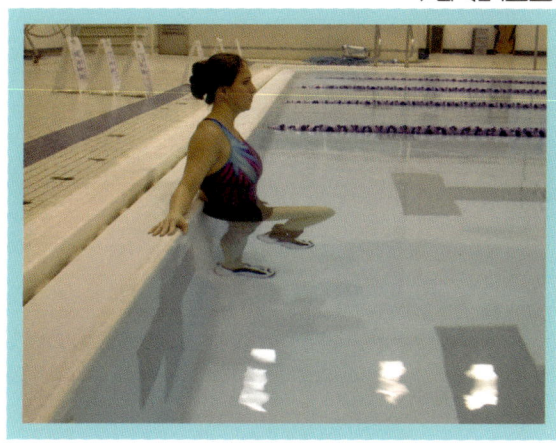

- Stand neutral/knee at hip level
- Knee stays stationary

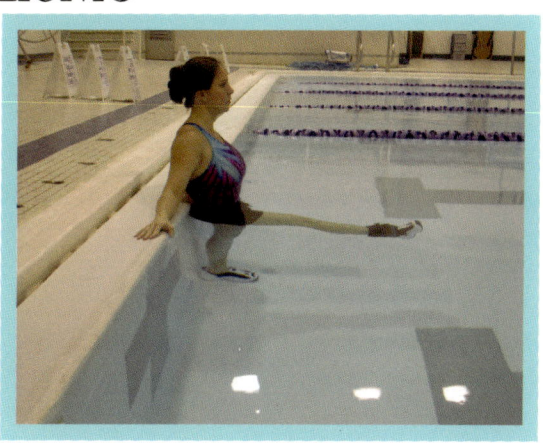

Push weight upward from knee/extending leg
Bend knee and pull weight back to start

AQUA TONE

SQUATS Target Muscles: Quadriceps/Glutes/Hamstrings/Abdominals

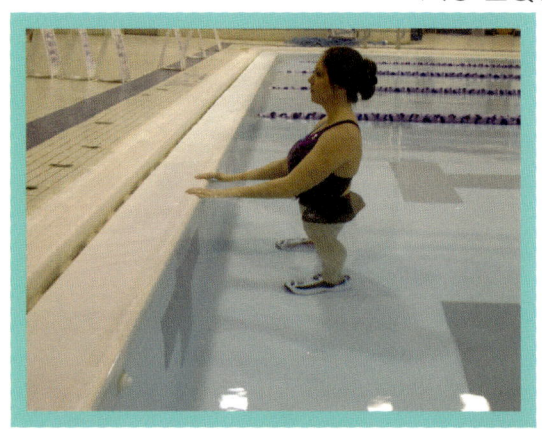

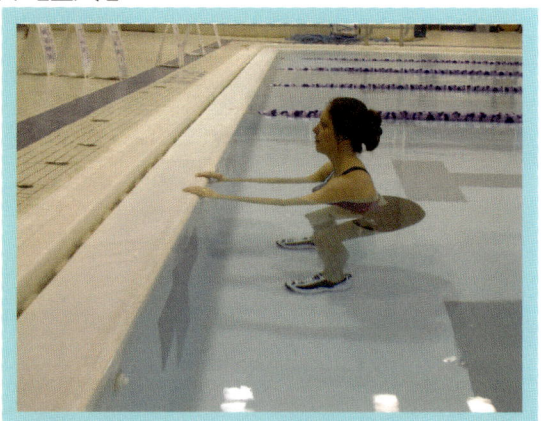

NO EQUIPMENT

WEIGHTS

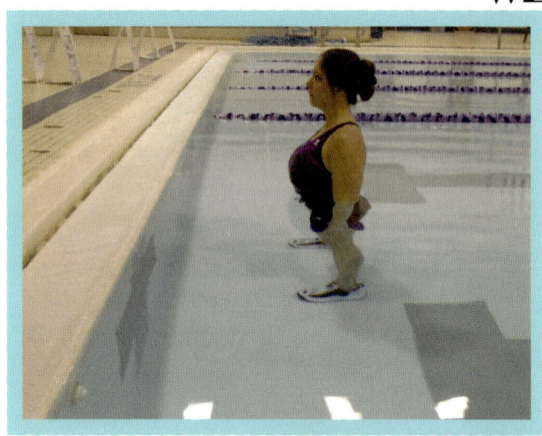

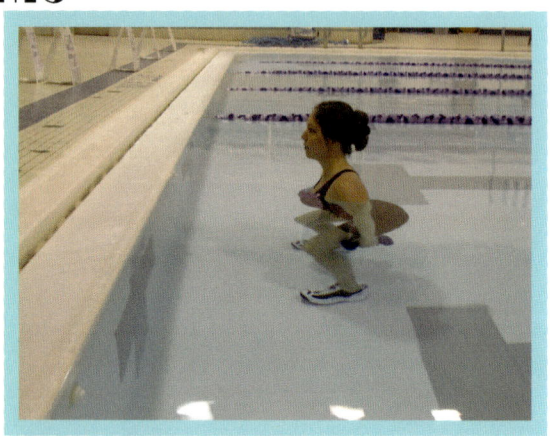

WEIGHTS WITH A FRONT RAISE

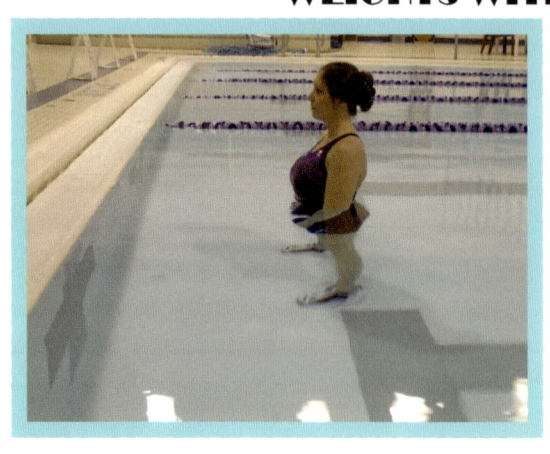

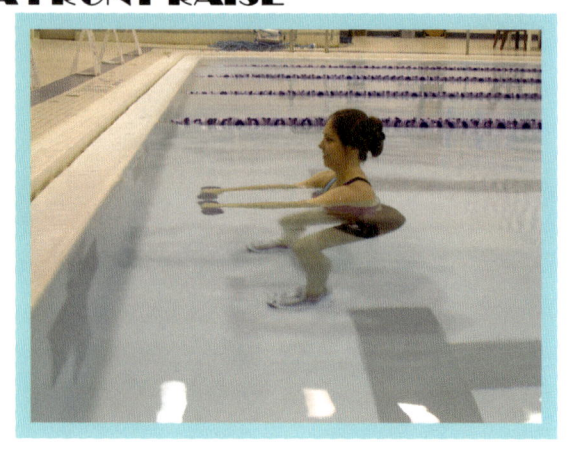

- Stand neutral
- Feet hip width apart
- Knees and feet pointing in same direction

Bend knees and squat down as if sitting in a chair
Bring thighs parallel to pool bottom
Push body up to start position

✓ **Keep knees behind toes in squat position**
✓ **Bend from the thigh joint/keeping back as straight as possible**

AQUA TONE

SQUATS (cont)

WEIGHT BELT

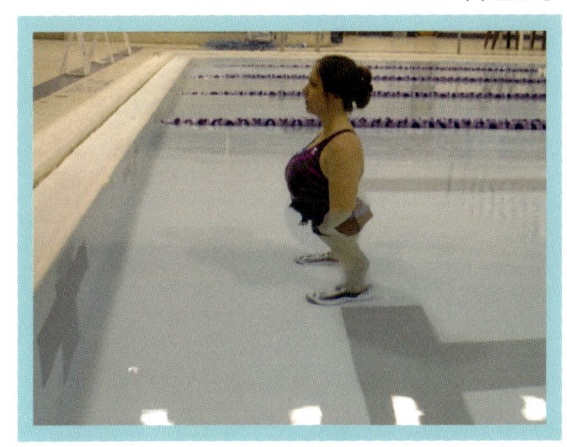

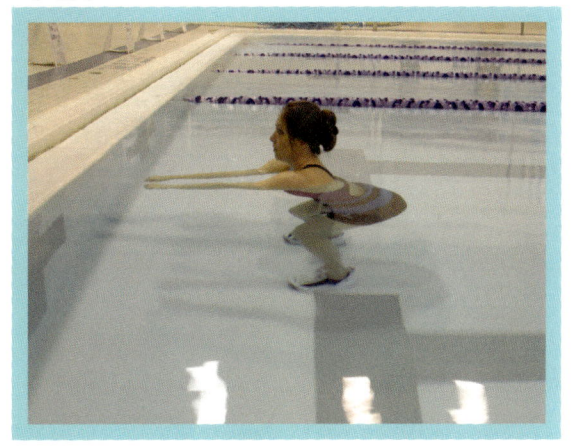

BANDS

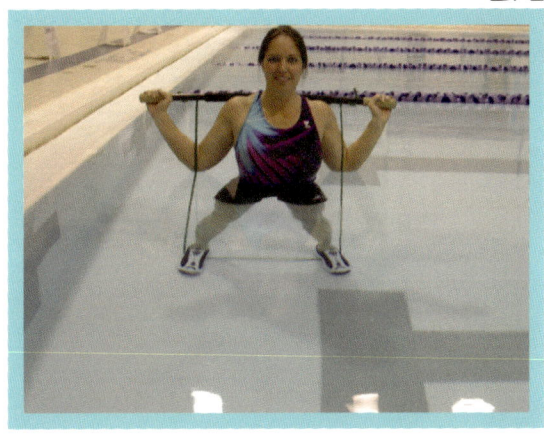

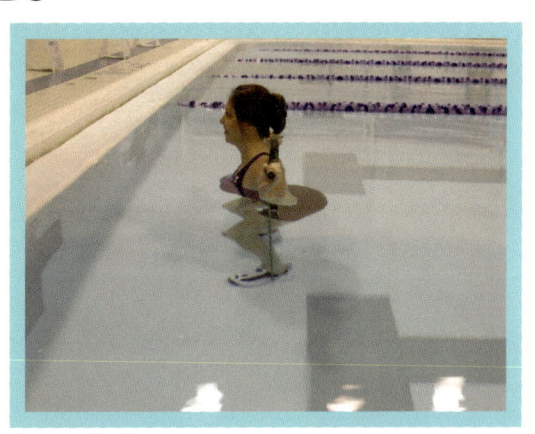

PLACE BAR ON TRAPEZIUS OR POSTERIOR DELTOIDS NOT ON THE NECK

- ✓ Follow instructions for squats on previous page
- ✓ Adding weight or resistance creates more work for the targeted muscles

AQUA TONE

SQUATS (cont)

WIDE LEGS

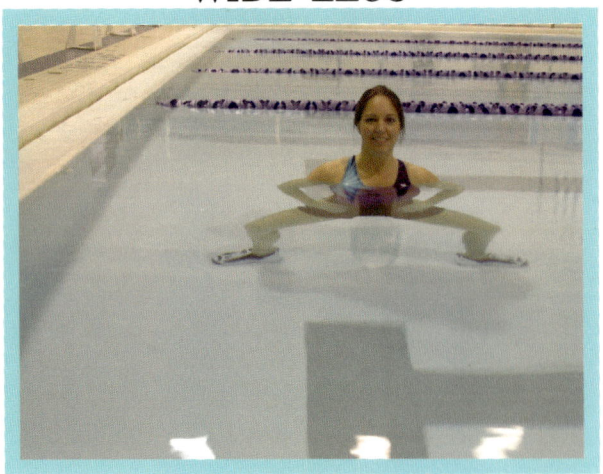

This position works all the same muscles but puts more emphasis on the inner thigh

✓ **Keep feet and knees pointed in the same direction**

STATIONARY LUNGES

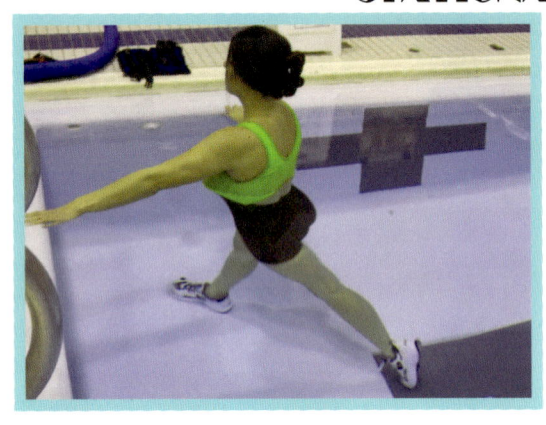

- Stand in a lunge position
- Knees and feet pointing in same direction

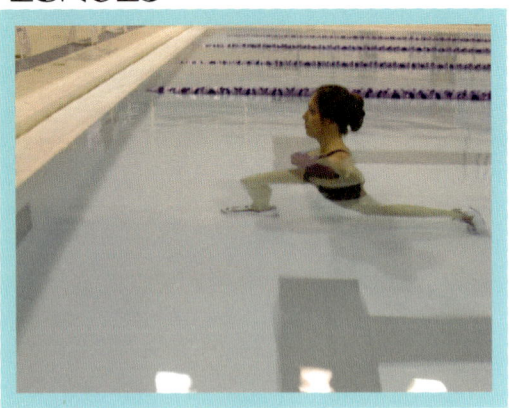

Drop rear knee down to pool bottom
Shift weight to front leg
Pushing through the heel back up to start

✓ **Perform intended repetitions on one leg then switch to the other leg**
✓ **Keep knee behind toes of front leg when dropping down**
✓ **Begin without weight and progress as in other squats with weight**

AQUA TONE

CALF RAISES Target Muscle: Gastrocnemius

WITHOUT WEIGHT

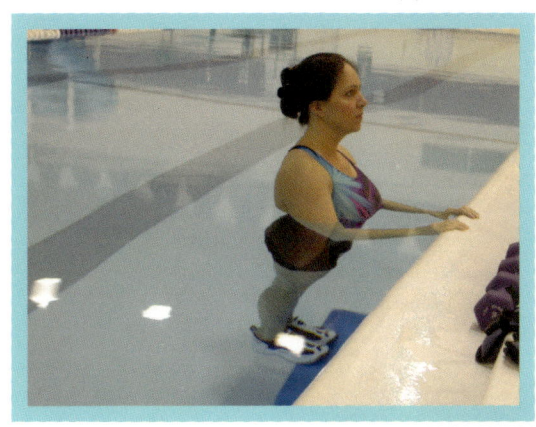

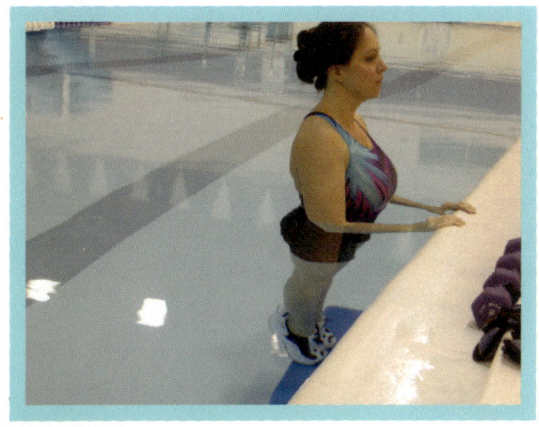

WITH WEIGHT

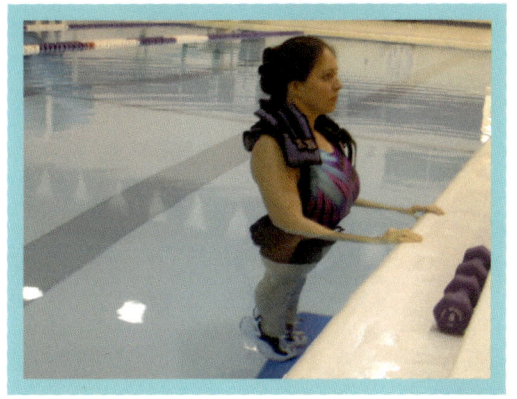

- Stand neutral
- Toes and balls of feet on step

Raise up as high as possible
Keep knees straight
Return to start position

✓ **To progress, add a weight vest or ankle weights on the shoulders for added resistance**

DO NOT ADD WEIGHT ON SHOULDERS IF SHOULDER OR BACK RISK CONDITIONS EXIST. INSTEAD, PROGRESS TO ONE LEGGED CALF RAISES.

ONE LEGGED

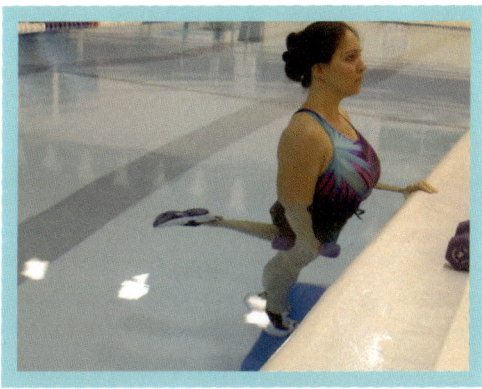

- Hold a weight in the same hand as the foot on the step
- Perform as in two legged calf raise

AQUA TONE

CRUNCHES Target Muscles: Abdominals

FLOATING

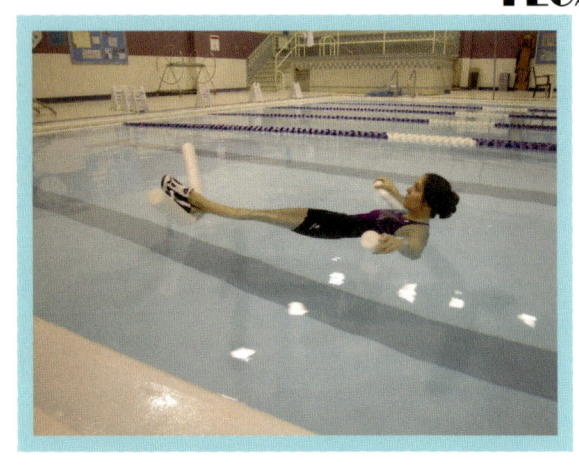

- Lying down with noodle under arms and feet
- Body completely extended
- Feet crossed

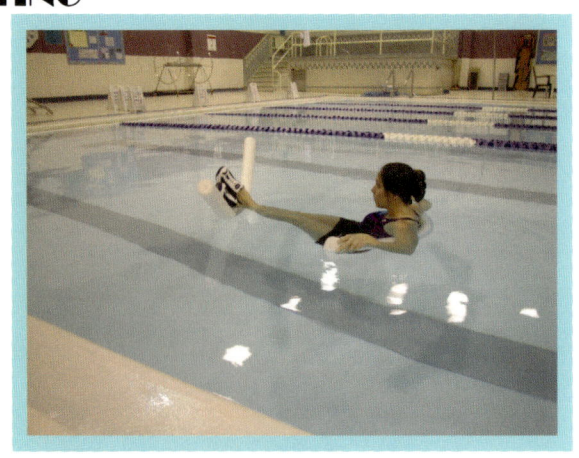

Bring chest toward feet
Exhale/Pull navel toward spine
Completely extend to start position

STANDING

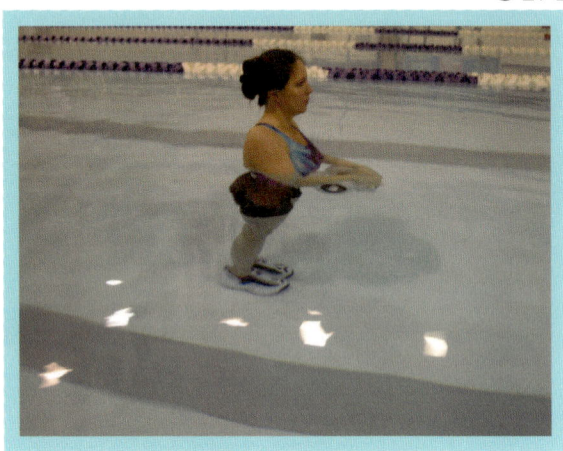

- Stand neutral/feet together
- Cross foam barbells and place at naval level

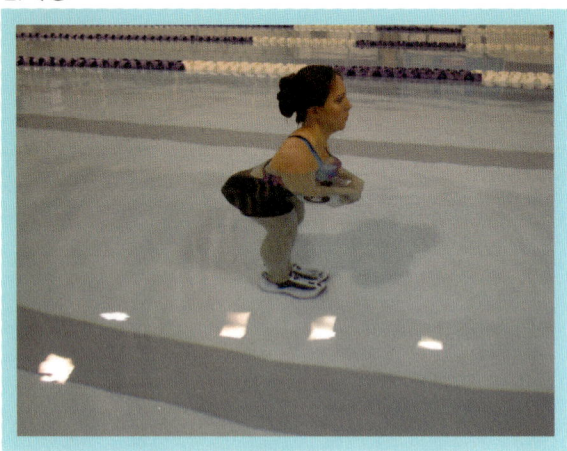

Bring chest toward feet
Exhale/Pushing down on barbells
Return to start position

✓ **Make sure to crunch (focus on pulling belly button toward spine)**

STANDING CRUNCHES ARE BETTER THAN FLOATING CRUNCHES FOR THOSE WHO HAVE NECK/SHOULDER OR BACK CONDITIONS

AQUA TONE

LATERAL BENDS Target Muscles: Obliques/Erector Spinae

WEIGHTS

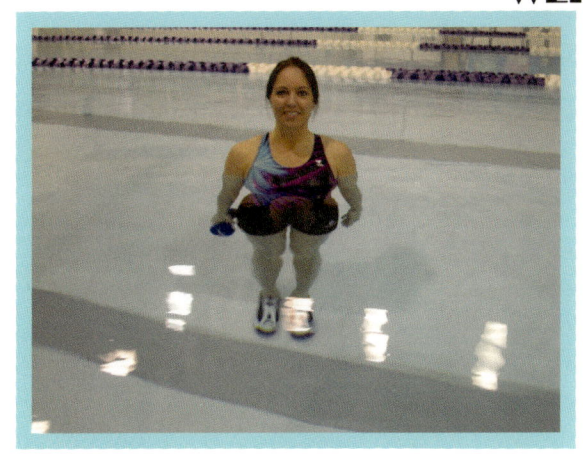

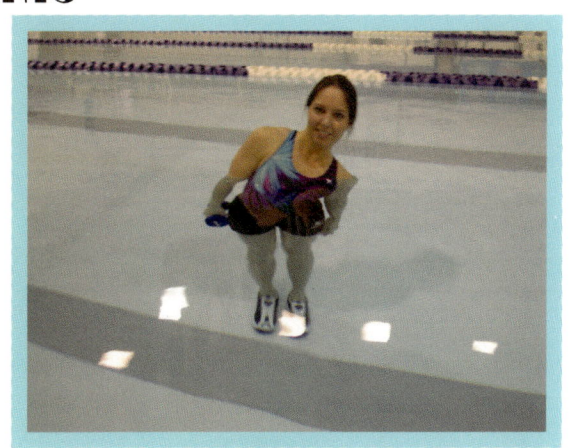

- Stand neutral/feet together
- Waist deep
- Tighten abdominal muscles

Bend the <u>opposite direction of the weight</u>
Run hand down leg to knee
Return to neutral

Perform intended repetitions on one side and then switch to the other side

FOAM BARBELLS

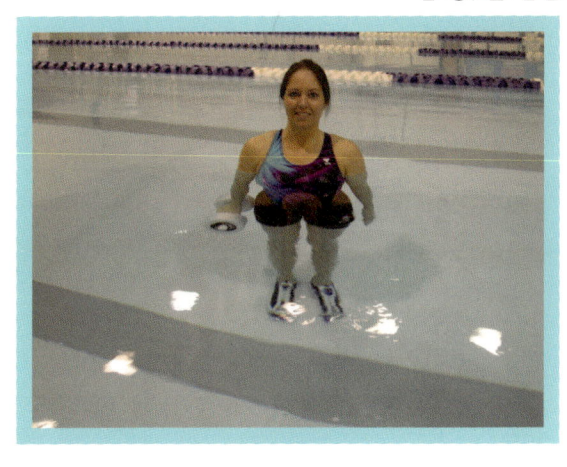

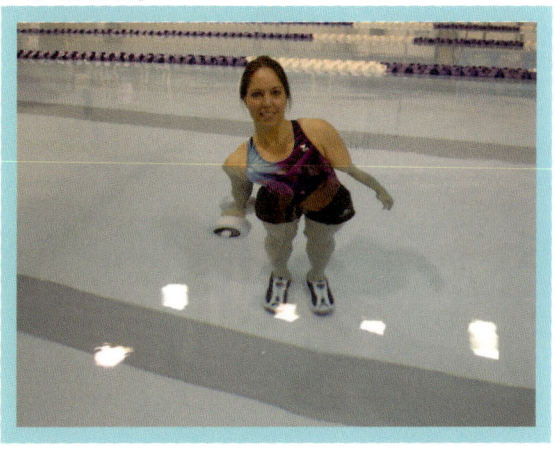

- Stand neutral /feet together
- Waist deep
- Tighten abdominal muscles

Bend in direction <u>toward the barbell</u>
Return to neutral

Arm holding the weight or barbell stays straight during bending motion

SAMPLE EXERCISE ROUTINES (These are only suggestions)

INDIVIDUAL

Level 1: Deconditioned, little or no resistance training experience, health conditions or injuries present. May need consultation with Doctor or Physical Therapist.

Start: No equipment, 2 times per week, 1 minute each or 8-12 repetitions

Exercises: Lateral Raises, Pec/Delt Flys, Bicep Curls, Tricep Pushdowns, Hamstring Curls, Quad Extentions, Adduction, Abduction, Floating or Standing Crunches

Progress: Gradually add equipment, increase frequency (3 times per week), increase intensity (work a little harder), increase time or repetitions.

Change it up: Add Front raises, Running Chest Press, Hammer Curls, Tricep Dips, Squats, Calf Raises.

Level 2: Some conditioning, some resistance training experience, minimal health conditions or injuries present.

Start: Light equipment, 2 to 3 times per week, 1 to 2 minutes or 12-15 repetitions.

Exercises: Lateral Raises, Chest Press, Compound Row, Bicep Curls, Tricep Pushdowns, Adduction, Abduction, Straight Leg Kick Back, Hamstring Curls, Quad Exentions or Quad Pushdowns, Calf Raises, Floating or Standing Crunches.

Progress: Increase level of resistance with equipment, increase frequency (three times per week), increase intensity (work harder), increase time or repetitions.

Change it up: Change type of equipment for the exercise, Add Front Raises, Hammer Curls, Tricep Dips, Squats or Lunges, Lateral Bends.

Level 3: Conditioned, recent participation in resistance training, No health conditions or injuries present.

Start: Medium resistance level of equipment, two to three times per week, 2-3 minutes or 15-20 repetitions.

Exercises: Lateral Raises, Front Raises, Shoulder Shrugs, Chest press, Compound Row, Bicep Curls, Tricep Pushdowns, Adduction, Abduction, Straight Leg Kick Back, Hamstring Curls, Quad Extentions or Quad Pushdowns, Calf Raises, Floating or Standing Crunches, Lateral Bends.

Progress: Increase level of resistance with equipment, increase frequency (3 times per week), increase intensity (work harder), increase time or repetitions.

Change it up: Change type of equipment for the exercise, Add Overhead Press, Bicep and Hammer Curl combination, Pulldowns, Tricep Dips, Squats and or Lunges, One Legged Calf Raises. Perform Super Sets, Triangles, Pyramids.*

GROUP CLASS ROUTINE

Warm up (5-10 minutes with movement)

Strength Training (50 minutes)

Equipment: Styrofoam Barbells (size depends on level of group or individual)

Exercises: Running Chest Press, Pec/Delt Flys, Tricep Dips, Bicep Curls with jumping jack motion.

Time: 1 minute each for 3 sets (Progress with increased intensity for each set)

Equipment: Noodles (Adapted if possible for choice of varying sizes)

Exercises: Adduction, Hamstring Curls, Quad Pushdowns

Time: 1 minute each for 3 sets (Progress with intensity and vary tempo (slow/fast) for each set)

Equipment: Free weights (if possible, choice of varying weight)

Exercises: Lateral Raises, Squats with Front Raises, Hammer Curls

Time: 1 minute each for 3 sets (Progress with increasing weight or intensity for each set)

Equipment: Regular noodles and or Styrofoam barbells

Exercises: Floating and or Standing Crunches

Time: 3 minutes

Cool down and stretching (5-10 minutes)

Individual and group exercise routines will depend on many factors including the type of equipment that is available, the number of participants, size and depth of pool, anchor points, differing levels of ability and health status. For Personal Trainers, the choice of exercises will depend on client level, goals, health status and available equipment.

"The greatest wealth is health."

Virgil
70 BCE-19 BCE
Roman Poet

AQUA TONE

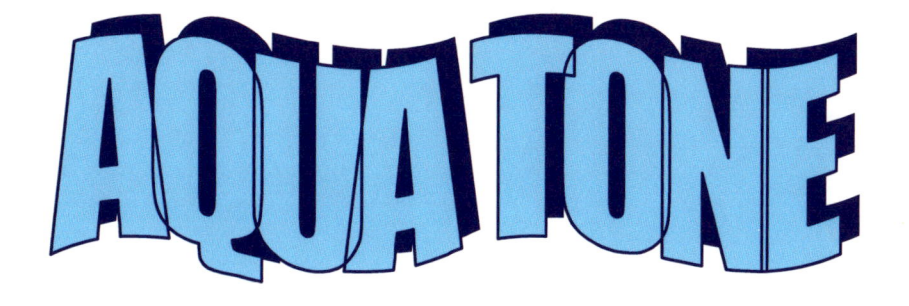

STRETCHING

STRETCHING

Stretching is an important component of any work-out routine. It can help prevent muscle soreness, reduce the risk of injury and promote flexibility. It is important to perform the stretch properly and to **hold each one for 10-15 seconds**. Avoid bouncing. Stretch between each exercise or at the end of the workout. Although there are many great stretches, I have shown only basic ones for each muscle group that might be worked in the Aqua Tone program. Hopefully, you have some of your own to add variety.

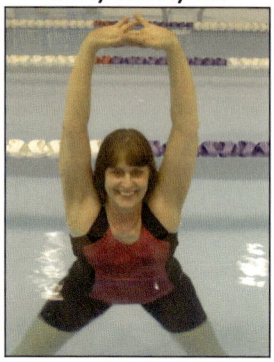

Arms/hands/abs
Clasp hands over head
pull hands upward

Triceps
Reach up with both hands and bend one down on to the back
grab the elbow with the other hand (this depends on flexibility)

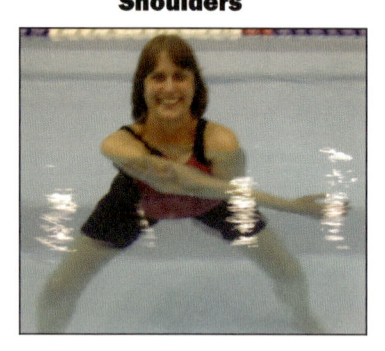

Shoulders
Reach under other arm
And pull shoulder close to body

Biceps
Pull gently downward on hand
of other straight arm

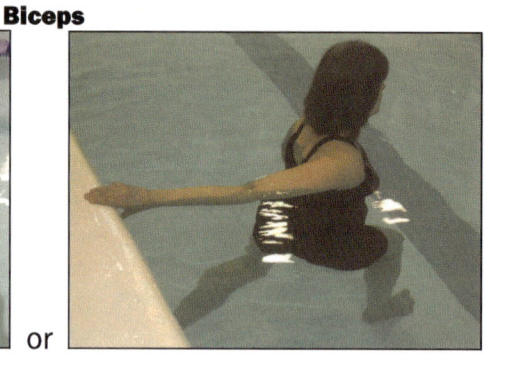

or

Face away from wall and reach behind
thumb down/same leg forward/lunge

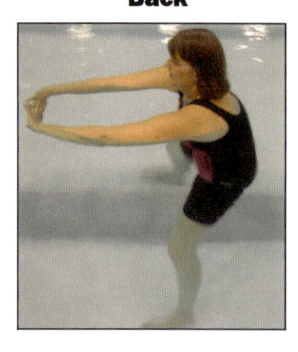

Back
Grasp hands in front
Pull forward/rounding back

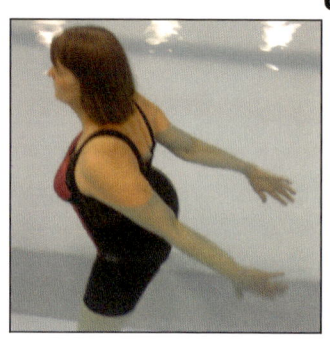

Chest
Reach behind body with both hands
If possible, grasp hands and pull back

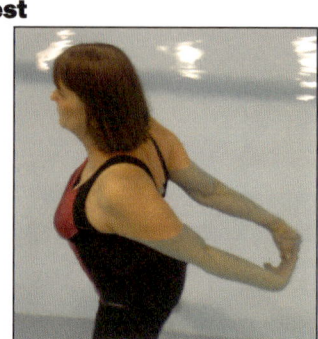

Quadriceps

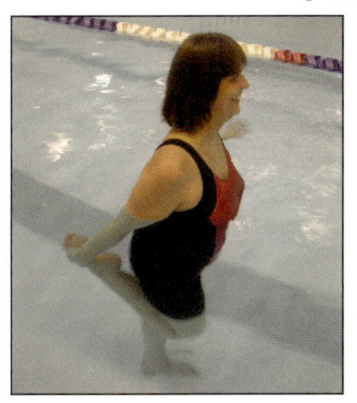

Hamstrings/lower back

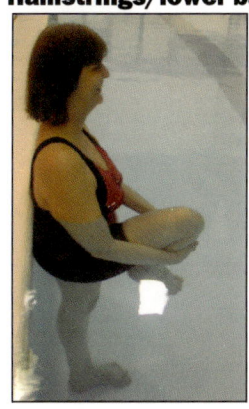

Grab foot or ankle with same hand. Keep knee facing down and close to other knee

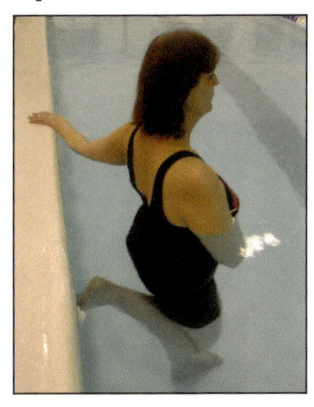

If grabbing foot is difficult, press foot against wall. Keep knee facing down

Bring leg up toward chest grab under knee and pull toward body

Calves

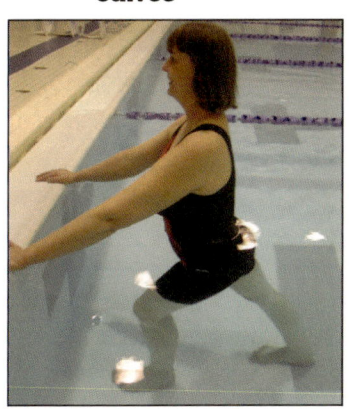

Inner Thigh

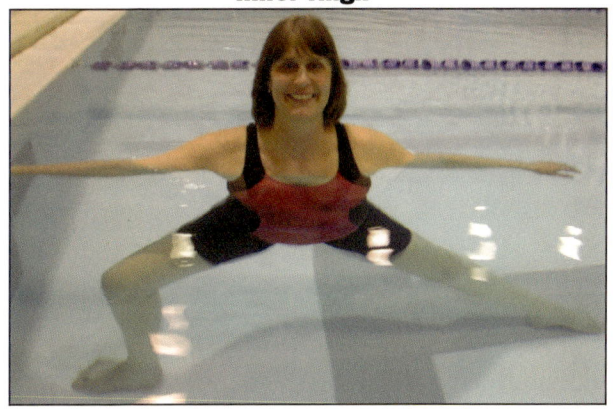

Bring one foot behind body press heel down

Lunge one direction straightening other leg. Keep knees and toes pointing in same direction

Hips

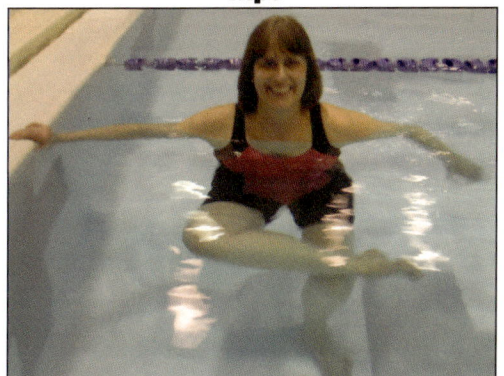

Place one foot on top of the other knee
Drop body down as if sitting in a chair

"Be careful about reading health books
You may die of a misprint."

Mark Twain
1835-1910
(Remember he was a humorist ☺)

REFERENCES

Aerobics and Fitness Association of America, <u>Personal Trainer Fitness Counselor Study Guide</u> (2002), Needham, MA

Aerobics and Fitness Association of America, <u>Aqua Fitness Home Study</u> (2002), Sherman Oaks, CA

Aerobics and Fitness Association of America, <u>Fitness Theory and Practice</u> (2002), Sherman Oaks, CA

Anderson, Bob, <u>Stretching</u> (2000), Shelter Publications, Inc, Bolinas, CA

Aquatic Exercise Association, <u>Aquatic Personal Trainer Manual</u> (2002), Nokomis, FL

Aquatic Exercise Association, <u>Aquatic Fitness Professional Manual</u> (1995), Nokomis, FL

Arthritis Foundation, <u>Arthritis Foundation/YMCA Aquatic Program Instructors Manual</u> (1996), Atlanta, GA

Bates, Andrea and Hanson, Norm. <u>Aquatic Exercise Therapy</u> (1996) W.B. Saunders Company, Philadelphia, PA

Delavier, Frederic, <u>Strength Training Anatomy</u>, revised Human Kinetics (2001), Editions Vigot (1998), Paris, France

Huey, Lynda and Forster, Robert, <u>The Complete Waterpower Workout Book</u>, (1993), Random House, New York

Rodriguez, Mimi, <u>Aqua Fitness</u>, (2002) DK Publishing, Inc, New York

Saunders, W.B., <u>Aquarobics, The Training Manual</u>, Harcourt Brace and Company Limited (1998), London

<u>Internet Sources</u>:

Bayer, Jeff, "Shock Your muscles with Supersets" askmen.com

DePuy Orthopaedics, Inc, "Strength Training and Weight Training for Arthritis Patients", allaboutarthritis.com

Quinn, Elizabeth, "Efficient Strength Training" (2006) sportsmedicine.about.com, New York Times Company

Sisco, Pete, "Training Opposing Muscle Groups" (2007) askmen.com

Waehner, Paige, "Get Out Of Your Rut – Changing your workouts" (2004) about.com/exercise

REFERENCES (con't)

Waehner, Paige, "Strengthen Your Core" (2008) about.com/exercise

Webster, Deborah, "The Neutral Spine", (2001) Wellbridge.com, Cambridge MA

Wikipedia, The free encyclopedia, "Weight Training" (July 2007)

Wikipedia, The free encyclopedia, "Resistance Training" (January 2008)

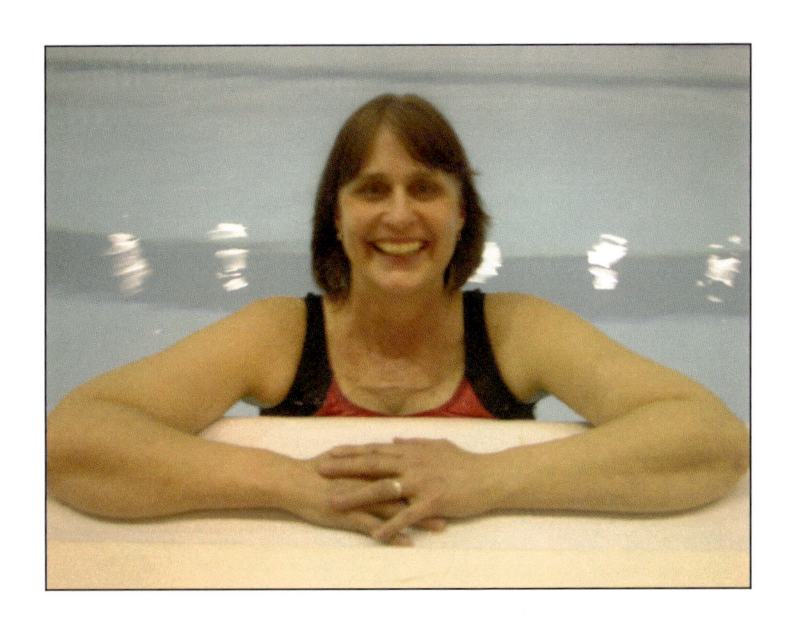

ABOUT THE AUTHOR

Patty Bowman has been certified with the Aquatic Exercise Association as an instructor since 1992 and as an Aquatic Personal Trainer since 2003. She is also certified with the Aerobics and Fitness Association of America as a land Personal Trainer since 2002. She has been a certified Water Safety Instructor and Lifeguard with the Red Cross since 1976. In 1983, she graduated from college with a B.S. in Recreation with a therapeutic emphasis. She has been employed with the Alaska Club/Fairbanks for 11 years as a swim teacher, lifeguard, water fitness instructor and personal trainer. Her main objective has always been to work with people in the water either by teaching skills, educating for fitness or providing therapeutic guidance.

ABOUT THE PICTURE MODEL

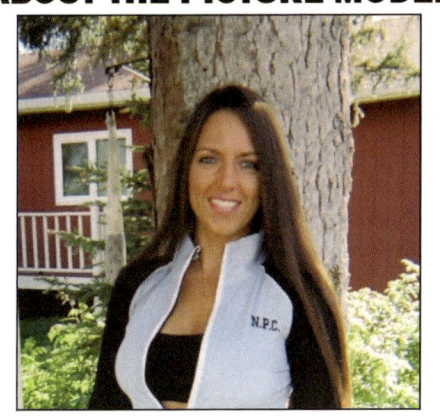

Sheila Bratten has been certified with the Aquatic Exercise Association as an Aquatic Fitness Professional since 2001. She is also certified as a stabil-a-ball and power attack instructor since 2004. She holds the 2004 title of "Mrs. Alaska, United States". Currently she competes as a national figure competitor with National Physique Committee.

CPSIA information can be obtained
at www.ICGtesting.com
Printed in the USA
2713LVUK00006B